4.99

VASECTOMY AND S
Making the rig

SUZIE HAYMAN is an ag
broadcaster. She is on the Bo,
Centres and a member of the N;
Family Planning Association. ..σ. books include
Hysterectomy (Sheldon).

CW00393333

Overcoming Common Problems Series

For a full list of titles please contact
Sheldon Press, Marylebone Road, London NW1 4DU

Overcoming Common Problems Series

Overcoming Common Problems Series

The Irritable Bowel Diet Book
ROSEMARY NICOL

The Irritable Bowel Stress Book
ROSEMARY NICOL

Jealousy
DR PAUL HAUCK

Learning from Experience
A woman's guide to getting
older without panic
PATRICIA O'BRIEN

Learning to Live with Multiple Sclerosis
DR ROBERT POVEY, ROBIN DOWIE
AND GILLIAN PRETT

Living Alone – A Woman's Guide
LIZ McNEILL TAYLOR

Living Through Personal Crisis
ANN KAISER STEARNS

Living with Grief
DR TONY LAKE

Living with High Blood Pressure
DR TOM SMITH

Loneliness
DR TONY LAKE

Making Marriage Work
DR PAUL HAUCK

Making the Most of Loving
GILL COX AND SHEILA DAINOW

Making the Most of Yourself
GILL COX AND SHEILA DAINOW

Making Time Work for You
An inner guide to time management
MAREK GITLIN

Managing Two Careers
PATRICIA O'BRIEN

Meeting People is Fun
DR PHYLLIS SHAW

Menopause
RAEWYN MACKENZIE

The Nervous Person's Companion
DR KENNETH HAMBLY

Overcoming Fears and Phobias
DR TONY WHITEHEAD

Overcoming Shyness
A woman's guide
DIANNE DOUBTFIRE

Overcoming Stress
DR VERNON COLEMAN

Overcoming Tension
DR KENNETH HAMBLY

Overcoming Your Nerves
DR TONY LAKE

The Parkinson's Disease Handbook
DR RICHARD GODWIN-AUSTEN

Say When!
Everything a woman needs to know about
alcohol and drinking problems
ROSEMARY KENT

Slay Your Own Dragons
How women can overcome
self-sabotage in love and work
NANCY GOOD

Sleep Like a Dream – The Drug-Free Way
ROSEMARY NICOL

A Special Child in the Family
Living with your sick or disabled child
DIANA KIMPTON

Talking About Anorexia
How to cope with life without starving
MAROUSHKA MONRO

Think Your Way to Happiness
DR WINDY DRYDEN AND JACK
GORDON

Trying to Have a Baby?
Overcoming infertility and child loss
MAGGIE JONES

A Weight Off Your Mind
How to stop worrying about your
body size
SUE DYSON

Why Be Afraid?
DR PAUL HAUCK

You and Your Varicose Veins
DR PATRICIA GILBERT

You Want Me to Do *What*?
A guide to persuasive communication
PATRICK FORSYTH

Your Arthritic Hip and You
GEORGE TARGET

Your Grandchild and You
ROSEMARY WELLS

Overcoming Common Problems

VASECTOMY AND STERILIZATION
Making the right decision

Suzie Hayman

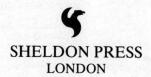

SHELDON PRESS
LONDON

First published in Great Britain in 1992
Sheldon Press, SPCK, Marylebone Road, London NW1 4DU

Vasectomy and Sterilization is a revised and updated edition of
Vasectomy and Sterilization: What You Need to Know, published by
Thorsons Publishing Group Ltd in 1989.

British Library Cataloguing-in-Publication Data
A catalogue record for this book is available from the British Library
ISBN 0–85969–657–X

Photoset by Deltatype Ltd, Ellesmere Port, Cheshire
Printed in Great Britain by Biddles Ltd, Guildford and King's Lynn

Contents

Acknowledgements

Many thanks: to Toni Belfield for her help, advice and suggestions; to Robin Ballard for the same and the practical demonstration (you *really* can't see the scars after the first year); to my Indefatigable Constant Reader and Companion who, thank goodness, never imitated Dorothy Parker, and to Phil for the funniest post-vasectomy anecdote I've ever heard.

Foreword

by Toni Belfield
Head of Information and Research, Family Planning Association

Increasingly, we are living in a consumer-orientated age – choice about many aspects of our lives and lifestyles is something we may tend to take for granted. This is especially true today: many assume not only that we are well-informed about subjects to do with reproduction, but also that the mystery and embarrassment that traditionally surround sexuality and family planning has somehow vanished. Sadly, this is not the case. The many thousands of enquiries to the Family Planning Association's information service show that the myths, misinformation and embarrassment remain and surround anything to do with sex, reproductive health or family planning. Why should this be? It is because the subject is not often discussed really openly or honestly – it is very often trivialized or simply swept under the carpet. The media's obsession with sex and reproduction results in an endless daily stream of information, which at its best is useful and factually correct – but more often than not presents a misleading picture. At its worst, it is sensationalist and full of mixed messages. So, while many of us are well-informed about the choice of family planning methods and their risks and benefits, considerable confusion exists because of the abundant contradictory misinformation perpetuated from various sources.

Nearly all of us think about, or use, a family planning method at some point in our lives. But how do we decide which method to use? How do we sort out fact from fiction? How do we evaluate what is safe for us? How do we evaluate what will be effective for us? Often it seems that family planning decisions are made by a system of trial and error, or simply trying a method a friend has used. For many of us, choice in some cases is not so much a positive one, but a negative one, in that the method *not* chosen is even more disliked than the method that is chosen. This seems a sad state of affairs in this day and age.

Sterilization – that 'final' step – is something many consider, many talk about and, to date, something three million couples in the

UK have actually gone ahead with. Any decision to be sterilized is a very important one, and should not be taken lightly. Whilst the surgical procedures for both male and female sterilization are relatively simple, there is a range of complex and emotional issues which need to be considered carefully beforehand. Not least of these is the implication which sterilization has for fertility and reproductive ability.

For all these reasons, I really welcome the revised edition of this book by Suzie Hayman. As a family planning professional handling many thousands of enquiries each year from consumers and health care professionals, I have long felt the need for a definitive guide on sterilization for consumers. As the decision to be sterilized usually (and ideally) involves couples, it is absolutely right that this book should cover male and female methods. It examines in depth the decision-making processes which men and women both individually and collectively need to make, as well as giving full and honest explanations of what to expect before, during and after a sterilization.

This book *does* sort out fact from fiction and provides the reader with accurate, up-to-date and, most importantly, objective information, so truly informed choices can be made – and made with confidence.

Toni Belfield

Introduction

Why sterilization?

Sterilization is an operation that leaves a woman unable to become pregnant or a man unable to make a woman pregnant. Fertility and potency – the ability to reproduce and the ability to make love – are areas of our lives that have tremendous importance and so exert considerable pressure on most human beings. For this reason, sterilization is a procedure surrounded by myths, fears and confusion. Perhaps surprisingly, it is nonetheless enormously popular.

Since the first recorded female sterilization in 1881 and the first reported male sterilization or vasectomy in 1894, a steadily increasing number of men and women all over the world have chosen this as *their* way of controlling their fertility. Now, well over 100 million people worldwide use it as the birth control method of their choice. One in three couples who use some form of contraception rely on male or female sterilization.

Sterilization has become particularly popular in the last fifteen years or so. As many women had a sterilizing operation between 1970 and 1980, for instance, as had done so in the preceding 90 years. Today, in Britain, as many as one in four married couples rely on it as their method. Some studies suggest that eventually an even higher percentage of couples may use surgery to put a final end to childbearing. In one American study, one or other partner in *half* the couples who were white, were married and were practising contraception, had been sterilized.

What sort of people are sterilized? Until fairly recently, this method of birth control had been used mostly by older couples with large families. A typical sterilization client might be in their mid-thirties with two or more children, have used contraception for some years but have had at least one unwanted or unplanned pregnancy or a 'scare'. Often, the other methods of contraception available have been used with a varying degree of success or have caused distaste or difficulties.

These are the facts, but they have often been interpreted in such a way as to make sterilization seem undesirable or suspect. It has been suggested, for instance, that sterilization, particularly vasectomy, is a 'blue collar' operation – a method favoured by people who prefer a traditional balance of power or who can't or won't use

1

other methods efficiently. Vasectomy, like using condoms, can be seen as giving the responsibility for contraception solely to the male partner. For these reasons, some people might not want to consider sterilization, on the grounds that it is déclassé or sexist, or it implies that you aren't capable of using any other method. However, if you don't see yourself fitting into any of these categories, or resent the idea that you might, don't reject sterilization until you have had a chance to consider further.

Many of the impressions you might have about this operation could be out of date or based on incorrect information. For a start, people in this country who have been sterilized come from every class, educational level and financial position. Increasingly, people who *are* being sterilized are coming from a wider range of age groups and have a smaller number of children than before. It may once have been true that opting for this operation was often less a matter of *choice* than 'an offer you can't refuse', either from force of circumstances or pressure from well-meaning professionals. Now, most couples who wish to be sterilized approach their doctors with their minds already made up rather than having the subject raised by a professional.

Many couples are shifting their perceptions about contraception and beginning to see it as a *joint* responsibility, no matter which of them is employing the method at the time. When the male partner makes it his business to remember when oral contraception should be taken, buys spermicide or fetches the diaphragm from the bathroom cupboard; when the female partner carries and puts the condom on her companion, it becomes less easy to divide contraception firmly into 'male' and 'female' methods.

But why has sterilization suddenly become so popular? The rise in operations is partly due to a change in the needs and attitudes of us, the patients or consumers. When contraception was a hit-and-miss affair, an unplanned pregnancy might have been met with distress, but it had to be accepted with a degree of fatalism. Improved contraceptive methods have led couples and individuals to *expect* control over their own fertility, and to look on pregnancies that were less than welcome as unwanted. This 'contraceptive mentality' means that many people are now able to plan their lifestyle and their families. And having made those decisions, the best way of making sure you won't have any accidents is to employ the most effective and least troublesome method of contraception, sterilization.

This trend could also be accounted for by a shift in the views of doctors. New, young doctors trained in an era which has seen birth control become available and free through the National Health, see nothing morally wrong in contraception in general or sterilization in particular. Instead of feeling that birth control is rather unsavoury and none of their business, or applying strict or paternalistic rules over who should be allowed to have it, most doctors have become positively welcoming and supportive. Indeed, the NHS (Family Planning) Amendment Bill of 1974, which provided for contraception to be available on the NHS, specifically allowed for local authorities to provide and support vasectomy services. Contrary to popular myth (a myth believed by the medical profession as much as by patients), sterilization has never been banned by law. However, various religions have considered such an operation contrary to their observance. The Catholic faith is still against it, but the Church of England allows it.

Being able to determine the size of one's family has always been given as a reason for seeking sterilization. The major change in the last few decades is that the average age of the requesters is now younger at the time of their decisions. Indeed, you could argue that the dramatic increase in the number of sterilization clients is really just a statistical anomaly. The actual number of people who would have had the operation at some point in their lifetime is unchanged; they just happen to be having them earlier, *now*.

However, there is plenty of evidence to suggest that a larger proportion of our population are using reliable methods of contraception, and that a steadily growing percentage of these are opting for sterilization. The greater the number of people who use and are satisfied with a method of contraception, the greater the opportunity for others who might not have thought of this method to hear about it and become interested. Furthermore, a new phenomenon has emerged: the individual or couple with no children who decide to stay child-free and who sometimes make that choice in their twenties.

Is sterilization a safe operation? When compared to its alternatives, it certainly is. An unwanted or even planned pregnancy carries a far greater risk to your life, health and your pocket than sterilization. As more operations are carried out and doctors become more practised and techniques are refined, the methods used to sterilize both men and women become safer and easier.

For sterilization to become a successful method, you do need to be clear in your mind what it is you *want* from it. Vasectomy was once offered as a cure for impotence and as a rejuvenating device. It can do neither in itself, but neither does it remove potency or promote ageing. The reproductive organs of both male and female have three functions: they can give pleasure, they confer gender, and they can allow reproduction. A sterilizing operation affects *only* the last and does so without changing the potential for the other two in any way.

Problems with sterilization are often linked, not to the operation itself, but to the decision that prompted it. Circumstances, misinformation and well-meaning medical advisers sometimes force people into a decision they can regret, giving the method itself an ill-deserved bad reputation. The most important aspect of sterilization *is* the decision. In order to make this properly, you need information on the operation itself and on what it means to you, and you will need room for thought and discussion. This book aims to give you the necessary information and to prompt thought and discussion, and in doing so to help *you* decide whether sterilization is the right option for you.

1
Decision-making

It took us ages to get around to getting my sterilization. We had both thought about it for some time, but with one thing or another never got round to talking about it. I asked my doctor a couple of times, but he wasn't keen and a friend put me off with all sorts of stories. I felt really confused about the whole business and when the doctor at the hospital suggested it I just sort of fell into it. I don't regret having the operation, but I do regret not talking it out properly. I still don't really feel that I know what has been done to me.

Jane S

When considering sterilization, the ideal 'order of play' is as follows. First, you, or you and your partner, will need to talk over your feelings and your views about the operation and the need for it. Singly or together, you would then visit a medical adviser, discuss it with him or her, then seek as much information as you feel would help. You would return for further discussion with your partner before going on to see the doctor who would do the operation. When you and your medical advisers are happy about your decision, you will go on to have the operation.

A sterilizing operation is certainly something that you need to *consider* rather than *accept*. The more control you feel you have over the situation, the happier you will be at the outcome. 'Being sterilized' is a very different event to 'choosing to be sterilized' and people who choose to be sterilized are far more likely to be satisfied with the result than those railroaded into it. If you are in the unhappy position of being advised to have a sterilization because of ill-health or risks to any children you may have, do try to weigh up the pros and cons carefully. Sterilization may seem the only sensible course, but if you feel pressurized into it, you may resent the need to be sensible! If you agree to be sterilized while you are rushed down a hospital corridor on your way to a Caesarean birth or just before having an abortion, the chances are that you will have bitter regrets.

In essence, what you need in order to be able to make a decision about sterilization that you can live with is:

- *Information* You need to have the facts about what sterilization may or may not do to or for you and to be able to understand how this could affect the way you see yourself and the way you get on with your sexual partner.
- *Discussion* You need to do a lot more than passively receive the facts. You need to be able to discuss your feelings with other people. Either people close to you, such as your partner, who will be affected by the sterilization; or professionals or friends who can be objective and who can help you sort out what you really want and what is really best for you.
- *Time* None of this can be done overnight. However urgent you think your need to get protection from pregnancy, try to take this particular step in a relaxed atmosphere, not with a sense of desperation.

If you are considering having a sterilization, at some point a doctor will be involved – after all, who else can do the operation? When it actually comes to surgery, you might expect the professional to have the final word on what happens. But before you get to that stage, when do you ask your doctor to become involved, and in what capacity? It is significant that as many as three in five people requesting sterilization had first thought about the operation over a year before approaching their doctor. For most of us, the operation itself might be a mystery, but by the time we get to the doctor the ideas behind it are already well thought out and rehearsed. Will your doctor take the initiative, by being the one to suggest that sterilization could be for you? How will you come to the decision to be sterilized, and what influence will you have over the type of operation you finally undergo?

Few doctors are actually trained, and not all are skilled, in helping their patients make choices. Many doctors still see their role as caring and paternalistic – they have the knowledge and come to the necessary decisions *for* you, rather than *with* you. This may be justified in the case of disease and treatment (although even this is now debateable) but far less so in the area of contraceptive choice. Sterilization, particularly for the male, is a quick and easy operation for a doctor. It is often seen as the ideal and final solution to the doctor's problems with a patient's difficulties in managing contraception. The doctor does not have to live with the result, you do. What is a few minutes chop, snip and stitch to a surgeon is probably the most important decision in your life and one you will have to live with for 20, 30, 40 or even 50 years.

The medical profession has assumed an expertise in discussing contraceptive choice because of the need for their surgical or medical knowledge or skills. In fact, if or when you need outside help, it is *counselling* skills you might need to call on to make your choice, and not all doctors are able to stop *advising* and to start *counselling*.

What is the difference? When somebody gives *advice*, the suggestion is that because they have more knowledge than you they have the right or the obligation to guide you, the less informed, along the route they know is best. When *counselling* is offered, this means someone gives you information and then, without steering you one way or other, helps you make up your own mind as to what is the best course for you. Your doctor or another may have what they consider to be good reasons to think that a permanent method of contraception would be of help to you. If you do not share this opinion, the result could be a range of emotional, sexual and physical problems.

Professionals may be invaluable in helping you come to a conclusion. However, it is vital that you recognize that this is ultimately your decision, and yours alone. The most important task is to face up to all the elements that might influence your choice and to order them in such a way that you can come to a realistic decision, and a decision that you can live with. Most of us tend to make choices in life – choices ranging from a new article of clothing to a marriage partner – with surprisingly little real thought. It sometimes comes down to a question of what is hanging on the rails today! But, with a decision that may alter your whole life, it would really be to your benefit that you use every means possible to help you, however silly some of them may make you feel.

There are various strategies that are particularly useful but that can seem odd if you are trying them for the first time. One of these is a form of play-acting that we call 'role-play'. In this, you and another person take it in turns to argue a viewpoint, in this case for and against one of you being sterilized. By rehearsing all the arguments, by listening to someone else advance them, and by listening to yourself taking different positions, you may find that your true feelings on the matter emerge quite clearly.

Another strategy is for both you and your partner, or you and a friend, to sit down with paper and pencil and to draw up lists. These can be headed 'Advantages' and 'Disadvantages' or 'What I know about sterilization', 'What I've heard', 'What I fear' and 'What I hope'.

A third strategy would be to find people who have been sterilized and to ask them for their impressions. If you asked among your friends or at work, you would probably be amazed at how many people would come forward!

As well as not feeling too embarrassed to ask other people about sterilization, try to put aside any lingering shyness at getting and reading as much on the subject as possible. There are various organizations that produce free leaflets that can be of help to your discussions, and you will find their addresses listed on page 95. Their job is to spread information, so don't feel inhibited.

Many of us find that when we visit a doctor or counsellor, we come out feeling dissatisfied. There may be so much to ask that we leave some vital aspect out. We may feel too shy to ask it all, or fear that we are taking up too much time. An excellent strategy to overcome this is to write out, beforehand, all the things we would like answered. As the discussion progresses, you can even add new ideas to the list. It may seem clumsy, ridiculous or over-formal, but it really does work. Not only does this aid your memory and your courage, but somehow writing questions down makes them less embarrassing.

Making the decision about sterilization is very much like building the foundations of a house. If you don't get this right, everything else may come tumbling down. The operation itself carries very little risk to your physical or mental health, either at the time or later. But *regret* at making the wrong decision can have drastic effects on both. If your foundation stone is laid firmly, the result will be extremely satisfactory. But you have to be sure. There is no shame in taking a lot of effort to make up your mind and then deciding that sterilization is not for you. You may feel silly at having gone to all that trouble finally to back down, but you would look far sillier if you went through with the operation and regretted it. Indeed, you can change your mind right up until the time they wheel you into the operating theatre itself. The doctors concerned would far rather you pulled out at the last moment, however much of their time you might feel you had 'wasted', than have you go through with the operation and regret it.

You can carry out these strategies on your own, but it often helps to have the aid of a professional who is skilled in such techniques. . You may find the idea of talking to an outsider about such an intimate area of your life is embarrassing or annoying. You may find the questions they ask intrusive, rude or even impertinent. You or your partner may even get downright angry at the prospect of having to discuss these things with somebody else, although most people find it is far less alarming than they had imagined. Instead, it can be very helpful. You may feel that sex is a totally private event that should happen with the minimum of planning and that our bodies should remain unseen and untouched by anyone other than our sexual partners. But professionals such as doctors and counsellors are there to help you put your needs and wishes into action. Allowing some intrusion, under your control, into your private life enables you to have the best health care and the widest possible choice in many aspects of your lifestyle.

If you find yourself getting angry with professionals when discussing sterilization, it might be worthwhile to take a deep breath and to consider what is going on. Are you angry because some jumped-up, arrogant official is trying to tell you how to live your life, put unreasonable barriers in your way and impose their own attitudes? Or are you angry because somebody is asking you to look clearly at motives and a situation that you know in your heart of hearts will not bear closer examination? It is obviously impertinent for a doctor or anyone else to demand that you go through time-consuming and exhaustive discussions when you and your partner have already done so yourselves and come to an adult and considered decision. But is it too much to ask that you at least demonstrate that you have done this?

Your family doctor would seem to be the person in the best position to help you, whether you are just beginning to think of sterilization or have made up your mind and just need information or an introduction to a surgeon. Most of us hesitate to consult our family doctors because we know that they simply do not have the time to give us the opportunity for relaxed discussion during a normal surgery. However, most doctors would be happy to give you a longer appointment for such an event, if you made a request explaining what you wanted. Alternatively, your doctor may suggest you see a trained counsellor, either at the surgery or somewhere else.

There are two ways you might regard your doctor when you are thinking about sterilization. You might see him or her as a gatekeeper or a colleague. In the gatekeeper mode, the doctor either obstructs or helps you along the way to your operation. The aim is to persuade, pay or fool your way past this obstacle to your purpose. The great danger in this is that you can become so caught up in the need to win this game and get past your doctor, that you lose sight of whether your best interests *are* served in having the operation. There is no advantage in lying your way through your discussions with a doctor or counsellor. The only person who can suffer by this is you. Of course, the doctor may set up such a relationship. You may find that asking too many questions about the operation, expressing any worries or unsureness may well find its way into your medical notes as a warning: 'obviously unsure – likely to change his/her mind – not recommended for operation'.

You are likely to end up with the best result when the doctor is happy to be a colleague in your decisions. In colleague mode, your doctor and you work together and neither needs to persuade or fool the other. It is worthwhile shopping around for a GP who *is* prepared to play this role. You do have the right to change your GP, without having to give a reason. Just remember that if you do it too often you may get a bad reputation.

Doctors often put sterilization requesters into one of three categories: 'nearly certain', 'probably OK' and 'be wary'. Most would be happy to recommend sterilization to individuals over the age of forty, to couples or individuals with large families, and to those with medical conditions that could make a pregnancy a severe strain on their health. Most would freely consider requests from the over thirties in a happy and stable marriage, from those with a complete family (usually accepted as two or more children well on their way to growing up) or from those who have tried other methods of contraception and found these difficult or unacceptable. Most doctors would fight shy of recommending sterilization to young couples, single people, couples with very young children or a baby, those with an unstable or unhappy marriage, divorced people, couples where one partner is very much older than the other, those with a handicapped child or one with a poor life expectancy, and women with severe period problems.

There are certain questions a doctor faced with a request for sterilization will want to ask in order to be able to help you. It would be sensible for you to consider and discuss these beforehand. This is not so that you can have your answers off pat, but because these are the areas you will need to explore to make sure the decision to have a sterilization is the right one for you. The questions can be summarized under the following headings.

Reasons for requesting sterilization

First of all, you need to consider *why* you want a sterilization. There are good and bad reasons. However, what we define as a 'good' or 'bad' reason for wanting sterilization has changed in the last decade. It would be fair to say that doctors, as the people who could grant or withhold a sterilization, have traditionally been a sort of moral filter over who could or could not get through to this operation. So a 'good' reason meant a socially acceptable one. Doctors would therefore consider it acceptable, for instance, to help a young, over-burdened, mother-of-many to cope with her growing children. In the early days of the establishment of contraceptive services in this country, the people involved in making birth control available had to fight hard to make it respectable. They did this by emphasizing the altruistic rather than the personal benefits. Using a method of fertility control was 'family planning', and the selfless reason for doing it was for mothers to space their families in order that they could be better parents – less tired and more healthy and able to give a good quality of life to their children and husbands.

Perhaps, as we near the twenty-first century, we can be a bit more truthful. We use birth control for these reasons, but we also use it so that we can enjoy lovemaking without regret, fears or apprehension. This, of course, is why we find talking openly about birth control so difficult – using it does imply that we have an active and enjoyable sex life. Using sterilization can be felt as the most blatant sexual declaration of all. In effect, you might feel that you are saying outright, 'We think our sex life is so important and fun that we are prepared to have an operation to make sure that we can enjoy it without problems.'

Doctors are involved with giving aid to the sick and some of them still feel affronted at the idea of using their skills to help their patients *enjoy* themselves. It is as if there is a conspiracy to pretend that the real reason we seek sterilization is for our health. Hence the insistence by some doctors still that only the 'deserving', such as over-burdened or less well-off families, should be 'allowed' a sterilization, and that it should not be given for 'frivolous' reasons such as aiding a good sex life. However, many consultants are now prepared to be far more open and few still observe the '120 Rule'. This rule was an informally observed understanding that the age of the mother multiplied by the number of children already in the family should add up to to 120 or more before a sterilization should be granted. For instance, a 25-year-old woman with five children or a 30-year-old with four children would be sterilized, but not a 27-year-old with three.

Increasingly, however, both doctors and men and women asking for sterilizations have realized that the key to whether someone should or should not be sterilized is whether it is truly acceptable or unacceptable to them. Thus, when you now consider whether you have a 'good' reason to be sterilized, what you should be looking for is not a reason that will satisfy your doctor, but a reason that will satisfy *you*. And the vast majority of doctors will be asking their questions, not with their own moral values in mind, but in order to find out whether you are really ready for, and happy with, this decision.

Is it because you and/or your partner have decided that your family is complete? Or is it that you hope that sterilization will do something *for* the relationship or for yourself? Do you hope that it will cure a flagging sex life? Freedom from fear of pregnancy can improve some couples' sexual relationships, but equally, removing the possibility of pregnancy can take away the spice. Or do you hope sterilization might damp down sexual demands you find over-whelming? Again, this may be so, but only if one or other of the partners involved is convinced that the operation could have this effect. Medically speaking, a sterilization operation does nothing to change your sexual feelings or sexual performance. If you feel you are getting too much or not enough, these are aspects of a relationship that need to be discussed and sorted out in their own right. A sterilization operation will be of no help.

In some cases, it becomes the choice because of worry over the possible side effects of other methods. Couples often start to consider sterilization when their family doctor suggests that the female half of the partnership should come off the Pill, or if an IUD has given difficulties and neither find the idea of barrier methods acceptable. Sterilization is then approached with a sense of desperation, being seen as the only method left that will have a degree of contraceptive efficiency. Sterilization can also be offered by the doctor, or chosen by you, if other methods have not given satisfaction. It is sometimes seen as a 'last chance' method if everything else has failed or if the couple concerned are not happy with other methods. Many of us also still see it as an end-of-childbearing-lifetime method and even feel that sterilization and the end of the potential for pregnancy can also mean the end of the potential for sexual activity. It is only recently that increasingly more people seem to see sterilization as just another option in a lifetime of contraception use – a lifetime in which many methods may have been appropriate at different stages and under different circumstances.

Sometimes an interest in sterilization comes about from a problem or weakness in a relationship. Couples may see sterilization as a sort of punishment or penance. A man may have a vasectomy because his partner has had, or has made him feel that she has had, a hard time managing birth control, or a difficult pregnancy or a painful childbirth. 'The Cut', and what he might see as the removal of his virility, can be viewed by both as fair payment on his part. In some cases, vasectomy is his penance for having had an extramarital affair. In other cases, when a couple has decided that the family is complete but the woman still feels in two minds about this, vasectomy is an 'equalizing' operation. If no more babies are 'allowed' because of finances or health, and she has lost her job of being a mother, then he is made to lose his job of being able to be a father.

Some people may consider sterilization as a political decision. You may have strong feelings about world poverty and over-population, and make these a part of your reason for limiting the size of your family. But, sterilization is a method of birth control that is significantly different from other methods. It cannot, at the moment, be taken up and put aside with ease. This means that it has more of an effect on your life and on your relationship than any other method. It is extremely unwise to seek sterilization for a purely external reason; that is, a circumstance or emotional state that may change. For instance, in some cases people have sought sterilization because they were unemployed and felt they could not afford another child. Or because their partner was depressed and could not cope with another pregnancy. When prosperity returned to the family, emotional stability was regained, or the marriage foundered and the sterilized partner remarried, another child became feasible and desperately wanted. So perhaps the most important question to ask yourself when thinking about sterilization is, 'If my life changed, would I still be happy to have been sterilized?'

The other options

By the time most people find themselves considering sterilization, they may well have come to the conclusion that all the other contraceptive methods are unacceptable. More than 40 per cent of couples seeking sterilization have had failures with another method of birth control. Think again! Are dissatisfaction or problems with contraception a good enough reason to apply for the 'final solution'? There are quite a few reasons why many of us don't give all the available methods a fair try-out and dismiss them without proper thought. Before you use surgical means to end any future risk of getting pregnant it is sensible to consider other options.

Not only should you look at the other available means of controlling your fertility, you should look carefully at what you *want* from a method of contraception, and what you have found unpleasant, difficult or unacceptable in the methods you have tried. Sometimes it is not the methods themselves, or even our application of them, that pose the problem. Often it is that we have approached birth control without having had the opportunity to consider fully what we want or need from it. For more on contraception, see chapter 2.

Is your age important?

Your age and your partner's age are likely to be considered important aspects of the decision to be sterilized. Of course, attitudes *have* changed. Ten to twenty years ago, sterilization would only have been offered to couples in their late thirties or forties with several children. As we near the end of the twentieth century, couples are opting for smaller families and making up their minds about the size of their families at an earlier age. This means, as we have seen, that doctors are likely to accept requests for sterilization in younger couples in their late twenties and early thirties. However, many may then want to look at the age gap. If you have a husband 15 to 20 years older than you, you may find your doctor reluctant to operate on you, although a vasectomy could be offered. The reasoning is that with a much older man, you risk being left a widow while still being in your childbearing years. You might wish to remarry and to have further children by a new partner.

Is your reproductive history important?

How many children and how many pregnancies you have had is important. The accepted idea is still that couples with large families are a better risk for sterilization than those with smaller families or no children at all. The idea is that if you have quite a few children, you are more likely to feel that you have completed your family and will have no regrets at taking the steps to ensure you have no more. This might be a questionable theory. It could be argued, for instance, that if you choose to have a large family, having children is important to you. To be deprived of the opportunity to have more, even if you *know*, rationally, that an even larger family is out of the question, might be damaging. If your self-image is of a Mum or Dad, and you derive most of your self-esteem from this image, sterilization may be a blow to your self-confidence, however sensible it could be to stop or limit your family. On the other hand, individuals who have only one or two children may not have as great a need to see themselves as parents and so might feel happier at being rendered surgically incapable of producing children again.

Traditionally, sterilization is not seen as an appropriate method for individuals or couples who have not had children. The assumption is that as it is 'natural' to have children, and everyone has them at some time or another, a child-free sterilized person will change their mind and regret the operation. The attitudes behind this belief need to be considered. Whether or not you are a good subject for sterilization will depend on how you see yourself. If you feel that your primary aim in life is to reproduce yourself, then clearly having a sterilization without having had children would be a very bad decision indeed. Even if your medical advisers suggested that sterilization was necessary for your own health, the health of your partner or because any children of yours would be certain of having terrible disabilities, an operation to render you unable to have children might still not be desirable. The advantage of reversible methods of contraception is that you can still see yourself as able to continue with these roles if circumstances changed. But if this is not an important aim in your life, sterilization may indeed be a good option, whatever your age or marital status.

Sterilization therefore is really only a good method for people who see parenthood as only a *part* of their lives, and a part that has various stages. If the role of parent of a small child is an aspect of life that you have been through and put firmly behind you, or do not see as relevant to you, you are ready for sterilization. If you still go misty-eyed at the thought of babies around the house – wait!

The age and state of health of your children are also important factors to consider. Just after a birth may seem a logical time to be sterilized, since you are in hospital anyway. It may seem a good time for a man to have a vasectomy too, as he may be thinking, 'I don't want to go through this again'. But again, waiting is advisable. Babies *do* die during childbirth or in their first few months of life. However healthy you are and however much care you took during your pregnancy, children can grow up with disabilities that shorten their life expectancy and you may wish you had kept the option to have another child. It makes sense to wait until your children are well on the way to growing up before lowering the boom. If your family has been structured around having and rearing two or three children, it may be both different and difficult to feel happy and relaxed if one dies. However *you* feel, your other children might be put under stress by losing a sibling and feel happier if another brother or sister could be produced. Children cannot be *replaced* as such, but you might want another child in its own right if something went wrong. Certainly you and your partner should consider your attitudes towards this before going ahead.

The length and stability of relationship

How long you and your partner have been together and how well you get on is also something to examine. Unless you are absolutely certain that you will not want to have any more children, under any circumstances, having such an operation before you are sure that this relationship will last, or when your marriage is rocky, is asking for trouble. The majority of requests for sterilization reversal operations come from couples who have separated or divorced and have new partners. It cannot be stressed too much that whatever you think or your partner says, having a sterilization will not cure any problems within the relationship. A good marriage may get better as a result; a bad one will get worse.

Even if yours is a longstanding partnership that you think will remain stable, you should still consider the *quality*, not just the quantity, of your relationship. Foolproof contraception has a way of throwing up conflicts and anxieties in even a satisfactory relationship, let alone a troubled one. It removes excuses and focuses attention. If you needed excuses, or were trying not to look too hard at how you get on with your partner, this can be extremely uncomfortable. This is relevant because how you welcome or react to a sterilization can often be affected by your partner's attitude. Not even a husband or wife can actually stop their spouse having a sterilization even though the result may be to deprive them of a mythical 'right' to have a child by you. This right does not actually exist in law. As with any medical procedure, consent to operate is given by the patient. However, disagreement within a marriage over something as important as this would be worrying. However sure you might be that *you* are making the right choice, if your spouse disagrees, the two of you could be heading for misery unless you talk it out.

Whose decision?

If you are contemplating sterilization, one important area to explore is whether this is to be a joint decision or one you wish to make for yourself. If the decision is a joint one, that is, you and your partner have decided *together* that your joint family is now complete, you need to consider the following. A joint decision can be affected by a change in the other person's attitudes or a change in your joint circumstances. For instance, if the two of you feel your family is large enough, but a child dies, would you want another? If your partner were to die, or your relationship ends, would you want a child by a subsequent partner? Or, if your partner changes their mind and suddenly puts pressure on you to have another child, would you agree to this? A joint decision necessarily rests on *both* sides of the relationship remaining in the same frame of mind.

A personal decision, however, can rest entirely on your own shoulders. If you feel that *you* have had enough of childbearing and that, whatever happens in your relationship or relationships, *you* will have no further wish to have children, you can make the decision for yourself.

If you feel that the decision is a personal one and you have decided to go ahead, then all that needs to be considered here perhaps is which type of sterilization is right for you. In a joint decision, you and your partner may wish to explore the pros and cons of vasectomy and female sterilization, and make a decision as to which method would be right for *both* of you. Depending on your health, emotional attitudes, or even childcare arrangements, you might find that either the male or the female operation turns out to be better for you.

17

ADVANTAGES

Female sterilization	Vasectomy
Instant effect.	After two negative sperm counts, patient *knows* he is sterile.
Depending on operation, rapid post-op recovery. Patient on her feet from within a few hours to 48 hours later.	Rapid recovery, patient able to leave clinic in a few hours or less.
Can be carried out as an out-patient.	Can be carried out as an out-patient.
Can be done under local anaesthetic, which has almost no risks.	Can be done under local anaesthetic, which has almost no risks.
Reversible operation can be successful in 75 per cent of cases, depending on the method of sterilization used.	If done fairly soon after original operation, surgery to rejoin the vas is easier than that to rejoin the fallopian tubes.
	Operation is easy, quick and safe to do.
Operation gives the opportunity to explore the pelvic cavity for any gynaecological problems.	

DISADVANTAGES

Female sterilization	Vasectomy
No way of knowing if operation has been effective.	15–30 post-op ejaculations are needed before man is sterile. Repeat visits for sperm tests are necessary.
Hospital stay of 12–48 hours.	
General anaesthetic has risks.	
Operation can put other organs at risk.	
Can create heavier, painful periods.	

You do need to consider the wider implications to *both* partners if one of you has a sterilization operation. One particular, eminent family planning expert has a favourite trick question he asks his students: 'How can a husband's vasectomy give a wife painful periods?' The answer is that she may find these returning if, when he has been pronounced safe after his operation, she goes off the Pill and only then remembers that heavy periods was one of the reasons for using the Pill in the first place! Unlike an hysterectomy, which will result in the cessation of periods, there are no hidden benefits from being sterilized for a woman. Periods will continue as before. Indeed, they may well become heavier and more painful as a result of the procedure (see chapter 5 for more details).

Which member of your partnership should have the operation? Both methods have specific advantages and disadvantages. The most obvious advantage for both is that it puts control of your fertility into your own hands. This can be appealing if you want such control, or frightening if you would rather not have such responsibility.

The advantages and disadvantages of male and female sterilization are shown in the tables above.

In this context, it might be worthwhile to consider your attitude to an 'insurance policy'. Would you find the thought of sterilization more attractive or less frightening if you *could* have second thoughts? Again, the traditional view is that sterilization *is* irrevocable and that even considering a change of mind is an indication that it is not for you. But is this so? In the case of vasectomy, there *is* a possible fail-safe in the form of sperm banking. The male partner can make a deposit of his sperm, to be kept safely frozen. Organizations offering this service are listed in the appendix. In the event of a change of mind or circumstances, this can be used for artificial insemination. The drawback is that artificial insemination is less efficient than intercourse in making you pregnant. Some 65 to 75 per cent of women will have a baby as a result of this procedure as opposed to 80 to 90 per cent using intercourse. Another way is for both of you to consider the question of reversibility in choosing which of you has the operation and which type of operation you opt for (see chapter 6 for more details).

The obvious question you need to ask yourself before having a sterilization, of course, is 'Will I regret this once I have had it done?' However, your answer may be a bit more complex than a simple Yes or No. Someone who has had their eyes tested and is recommended to use glasses may regret seeing the optician, but understand and accept the sense of taking steps to protect their eyesight. You might have passing moments of regret and doubt over not having further children. But, in the final analysis, will you feel you have made the best move for yourself and those around you? And given the same circumstances, would you make this same decision again? If the answer to *that* is Yes, then perhaps sterilization *is* for you.

Case histories

Mike's and Tina's story

Mike and Tina were married while both were still in their teens – he 18 and she 17. Tina was pregnant with their first daughter, and by the time she was 21 they had three children. Tina was unhappy about being on the Pill. 'You hear of all these side effects,' she says, 'and I don't want to get fat or die of a heart attack.' Mike refused to use condoms and said he could feel a diaphragm – a method that Tina also found unpleasant and troublesome. Tina's doctor had a busy practice and she always felt that he thought her a nuisance – they never had time to discuss methods. It was just a case of 'Well, try this and come back if it doesn't work.' After three children, one miscarriage and one abortion, it seemed that none of the usual methods of birth control *were* going to work. Tina's doctor eventually suggested sterilization, saying that in spite of the fact that she was only 24 at the time, having three children did mean her family was complete.

Tina saw the hospital consultant, said that she did want the operation, that she and Mike had talked it over and were agreed. Yes, her marriage was stable and happy and, yes, she did accept that the operation was irrevocable.

A year after the operation, Tina saw a new doctor at her surgery and the real story came tumbling out. Mike and she had separated. Their 'discussions' had consisted of Mike saying, 'If you don't get your tubes tied, I'm leaving.' Far from being happy and stable, their marriage had always been uncertain. She now felt less of a woman and was bitter and resentful. She had felt forced into lying her way through the discussion with the hospital doctor in an attempt to stop her marriage breaking up. Her operation had not had this effect. Tina thought that three children were quite enough to be going on with, but she also felt that any future partner would not be interested in her if she couldn't give him a child of their own. 'I just wish I had spoken up at the time. They did ask me if I was sure and I suppose I was in a way – but of the wrong things. I was sure that I had to do what Mike said or he'd leave me. That wasn't a good reason to have the operation, was it?'

Pete's and Hilary's story

Pete and Hilary first thought about sterilization when a friend of theirs had a vasectomy. The friend had been delighted with the result and impressed quite a few of their other friends with how much simpler it made his sex life. Hilary was less keen because she hated hospitals and didn't like the idea of either of them having an operation unless it was really necessary. However, Pete made a point of getting hold of a book from the library and he also wrote off for leaflets on the subject. They found themselves talking about it quite a lot. Eventually, Hilary agreed to go with Pete to their doctor to talk it over. Pete had seen this visit as being no more than a rubber stamp. He expected the doctor just to send them on to the hospital. When the doctor started to ask some fairly searching questions, Pete got very annoyed and said the doctor was just being obstructive. After a bit of an argument, he stormed out.

The matter rested until Hilary took their youngest child for a tetanus injection and the doctor made a point of apologizing for upsetting Pete and explaining why he had felt it necessary to talk the matter over carefully. He pointed out that Hilary *had* had misgivings which Pete wasn't really allowing her to think over. He said he felt that if they couldn't at least bring these into the open and went ahead with the operation, Pete might be happy with the result but Hilary may end up being worried and resentful. When Hilary explained all this to Pete, he had to admit that a lot of his anger had been because he was trying to rush Hilary into a decision. 'I suppose I thought that if I went ahead and had it done, she'd come round and be happy. But thinking about it now, I know that it would have had the opposite effect.' In the second consultation with their doctor, Hilary and Pete were both able to put their points of view and Hilary found herself much happier about the idea of one of them having the operation. They decided that a vasectomy would be the best option and this was arranged soon after.

2

The alternatives

> I'd used the Pill ever since I was a teenager and when my doctor told me I had to come off I was devastated. The idea of fiddling about with bits of rubber and creams really put me off. It had been so easy for all these years that I really did feel that one or other of us being sterilized was the only thing I'd accept.
>
> Vicky M

Why sterilization? A reason often given for choosing this method of birth control is that the family is complete. This is, however, an argument for using contraception, not a sufficient reason for picking a particular *type* of method. However, sterilization seems the logical choice when your mind is made up, since it is considered to be the most effective method.

Not only are the other available methods seen as being less effective than sterilization, they are also often felt to be less acceptable. The Pill may be felt to have too many side effects, the diaphragm to be unpleasant and the condom unsafe. With the exception of the IUD, all have to be remembered and used regularly.

However, dissatisfaction and difficulties in using a method continuously or effectively often have nothing to do with any failing in the method itself. Frequently it is our attitudes and what we expect from the method that cause problems. Many of us allow ourselves to be burdened with unsuitable birth control and grow unhappy with it because very little *real* choice has been made. If your choice of contraception is to be right, you need to ask yourself, 'What do I want from a method of birth control?' Before you take the irrevocable step to end your fertility, it is absolutely vital that you look at sterilization and every other method of contraception in the light of this question.

The main purpose of birth control or contraception is to prevent pregnancy, or so we assume. For this reason, when we talk about the subject, the most important aspect of each method is felt to be its efficiency. The question, 'What is the *best* method?', is understood to mean 'Which has the lowest pregnancy rate?' Drug companies sponsoring research into new methods, doctors prescribing them and consumers asking for them all talk about the percentage efficacy rating of each. This is usually measured in 'woman years' – how many women would fall pregnant using this method if 100 of them used it for a year. The nearer you get to the 0 per cent rating, the better the method. If you have had problems with contraception or it is important to you not to have another pregnancy, sterilization may be seen as the obvious solution. But is this really the way to see contraception? *Is* protection against pregnancy the only or the most important factor that concerns us?

When you look at the way most of us actually behave, it becomes clear that for both men and women prevention of pregnancy may *not* be the only important aspect of a contraceptive method. The advantage that is most often talked about for sterilization is its efficiency. However, for many doctors the reason they recommend it is that their patients cannot inconvenience *them* by forgetting, losing or refusing to use the method they have so conscientiously prescribed. For the consumer, the main advantage is that we can get on with the real business of having enjoyable sex without being interrupted.

But there are some real disadvantages to this once you recognize that stopping you getting pregnant is not the only way a method of birth control affects you other than simply preventing a pregnancy. Unlike the Pill, sterilization cannot lessen painful or heavy periods. Unlike the sponge or condom, it cannot contain or soak up sperm and so prevent you from having to sleep in the damp patch.

What most of us would like from a method of birth control is something that, at the very least, does not interfere with our sexual pleasure or, at the very best, actually increases it. When we see our family planning doctor for contraception, however, very few of us would dare to mention concerns like these. It is almost as if we must pay for our pleasures by having to put up with a method we don't quite like. Complain, and we may be told that we are neurotic or that our relationship is clearly in trouble.

Complaints about birth control *can* have a shaky foundation. The ability to have or cause a pregnancy is felt by many of us to be a vital part of our self-image. If we feel guilty about our sexual desires or find them alarming we may only be able to be passive about sex. The use of contraception means having to say, each time we pick up a cap or Pill, 'I'm planning to have sex.' This may be difficult. If we find one method unpleasant and another impossible to use, it may be because we find it difficult to come to terms with our own sexual feelings or our guilt about them.

Sometimes, dissatisfaction with a method, or refusal to use one, is a statement about the sexual partner. Some men and women use birth control – or the lack of it – to have power or control over their partner's or even their own sexual desires. An insecure man may insist on his using the sheath or withdrawal or having a vasectomy in the belief that his wife cannot safely take a lover. Condoms can be mislaid or withdrawal left to the last moment so that he can have the accident-on-purpose and keep her 'barefoot and pregnant'. By not using a method, the insecure woman who finds no pleasure in sex can always reject advances on the grounds, 'It's not my safe time'. In many cases, difficulties with birth control *are* the sign of deeper problems.

But this is not always the case. When a particular reaction is consistent, it is time to consider whether it is the label of 'neurotic' that is wrong, rather than the behaviour itself. At the moment, we tend to have rigid assumptions about birth control. We believe that when a contraceptive method fails it is because users are being irrational or lazy or stupid. We assume that the answer is to make it more efficient and foolproof. But few researchers consider finding out *why* people find methods unacceptable, *what* we find unacceptable and *why* these factors should be more important than the fear of pregnancy.

Above all, contraception is seen in terms of long-term planning. 'If I use a sheath/cap/Pill now, I'll be glad in nine months time when I won't have another mouth to feed.' But who thinks like this in the middle of making love? You make love because you want to feel pleasure, show love or share sensation *now*. Unless sex is happening because a child is wanted, what may happen afterwards is hardly considered at the time. Uppermost in lovers' minds are immediate emotional or physical needs. Sex makes us feel good, lets us show affection and allows us to feel masculine or feminine. That is why the immediate and certain emotional or physical drawbacks of a birth control method become so much more important, *at the time*, than the future possible drawbacks of unwanted pregnancy. If the method is unpleasant or detracts from your fun, or makes you fear for your health, one of two things is likely to happen. Either you will not use it or you will find that your concern or distaste spoils all enjoyment.

Your sexual partner's attitude towards your method of contraception is as important as your own. You may sabotage your own successful use of a method by being ambivalent towards its use.

Your partner's hostility to a method you find acceptable can be just as devastating. Women can find their lover's use of a condom insulting or laughable and men can find the use of a diaphragm distasteful or excluding. The other person's use of birth control can also be seen as a threat to your femininity or masculinity and potency. A high failure rate has been found to go hand in hand with the objection by a partner to a particular method or general use.

You have to go through quite a complex process of decision-making before getting and using birth control. First, you have to admit to yourself that you *are* having sex and risk pregnancy. If you are inhibited or embarrassed about your sex life, this in itself may be hard. Some of us prefer to believe that sex is not something we decide to do – it just happens and we 'can't help it'. At the same time, the potential user must be able to accept that he or she *can* take control of their own life. To many people, life happens *to* them and they view their existence and any possibilities of pregnancy with a certain fatalism.

Even if it is accepted that the risk is real and could be avoided, the pros and cons of using or not using contraception have to be weighed up. The drawbacks of unplanned or unwanted pregnancy may seem obvious. There will be an extra mouth to feed, you may lose earnings or a chance to finish your education, you may find your social life suffers, and if you are young or unmarried people may well disapprove. But against that can be set the *advantages*. Parenthood gives you status, attention and someone to love and be loved by. A pregnancy will prove the maturity and the masculinity or femininity of the parents and test a relationship. Most important perhaps are the costs of using a method of birth control. Contraception may prevent pregnancy, but many people feel that contraception is embarrassing and troublesome to obtain, and that most methods are unpleasant or inconvenient to use. A common belief is that many methods get in the way of what the majority of people consider to be the real business of sex, which is spontaneous pleasure with no after effects. To many, the cost of contraception is too high.

The Pill was welcomed as a major development over 30 years ago. But 30 years later we are able to see it in a different perspective, warts and all. We now realize that oral contraception should be viewed as just one more method to be chosen from a range of equally valid options. The only problem is that too many doctors and scientists and too many users see the Pill as the top of the range

– the 'ideal' towards which all present and any future methods must aspire. The fact that the Pill is *almost* 100 per cent effective, almost entirely free from mess and bother and certainly divorced from the sexual act, means that we have set up efficient, mess-free and intercourse-independent contraception as our goal. And if, for some reason, this particular method cannot be used by us, the next most obvious method is sterilization.

If you are considering sterilization, the chances are that either:

- Your doctor has advised that you come off the Pill and you are reluctant to use a less effective method.
- You are worried about the side effects associated with your present method.
- You find all the other methods alarming or unattractive.

However, before you turn your back forever on the other methods, you need to consider whether your fears of their side effects or their inefficiency are justified, and whether they really are as cumbersome and difficult as you imagine or remember. So, first, let us look at how a pregnancy is started before going on to look at the methods to prevent this happening.

Inside the pelvic cavity, squashed between the coils of the bowel and the bladder, lie a woman's reproductive organs. These consist of two plum-sized and shaped glands called ovaries, and a pear-shaped and sized flexible bag called the uterus or womb. This lies stem end down, the stem being the cervix or neck of the womb that sticks out into the vagina. The vagina is the stretchy tube that is the sex or birth passage – the opening between a woman's legs. At the other end of the uterus there are two tubes that curve round inside the pelvic cavity, embracing the ovaries. These are the fallopian tubes.

Women are born with millions of potential egg cells in their ovaries. At puberty, around 200,000 of these potential cells, called follicles, remain. Around 400 might develop fully during a woman's childbearing life. From puberty until the menopause, a complex series of chemical signals occur each month to ready one of these cells for pregnancy. These chemical messengers or hormones are produced by various glands in a woman's body and they drive what we know as the menstrual cycle. On the signal from the hypothalamus, which is a part of the brain, and the pituitary gland at the base of the brain, ten to twenty egg cells will start to mature each

27

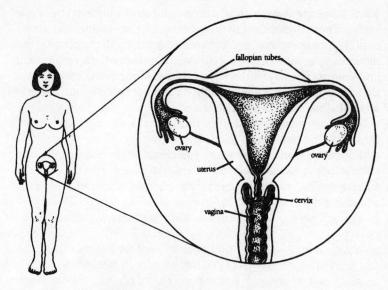

Figure 1 Female reproductive organs

month. As well as bringing these cells to ripeness, the ovaries send out their own chemical messages to the uterus. These trigger the endometrium or lining of the uterus to thicken and grow in preparation for a fertilized egg.

When one of the follicles is ready, it will burst open and an ovum or egg will be released from the ovary and be wafted on fluid in your pelvic cavity towards, and then down, the fallopian tube. This is called ovulation. Each ovary usually takes it in turn to release an egg. If sperm is not encountered at the right time in the journey from ovary to womb, the egg will not be fertilized and will be washed out of the body in the normal flow of fluid. The journey takes around seven days and an egg must meet up with sperm in the first 24 hours for a pregnancy to start. If it does, the male cell and the female cell will combine and the resultant bundle of cells, called a blastocyst, will continue down to the womb and implant in the womb lining. If the endometrium is not receptive or hormone levels are at the wrong stage, the egg will be rejected.

The male contribution, the sperm, is also triggered by action of the hypothalamus and the pituitary gland at the base of the brain. In men, the hormones produced act on the testes, the two glands suspended outside the body in the scrotal sac underneath the penis.

From puberty, these glands manufacture sperm which are made anew continuously. Sperm is produced in enormous quantities inside each testicle in a complex system of tubes called seminiferous tubules. They pass from these through a network – the rete testis – into the epididymus. This is a long, coiled tube which in turn passes the sperm into the channel called the vas deferens. Each vas leads to a small gland called a seminal vesicle. The two channels come together in the prostate gland. Here, sperm is mixed with a liquid called seminal fluid which passes out via the urethra down the penis to the outside world. Each male ejaculation will contain around 300 million sperm. However, 98 per cent of the teaspoon of liquid that is an ejaculation is actually seminal fluid – the fluid which nourishes and protects the sperm on its journey.

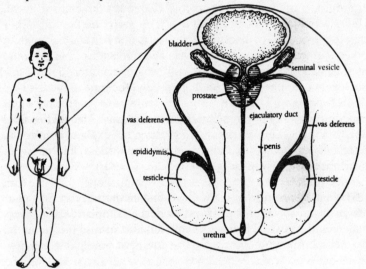

Figure 2   Male reproductive organs

Sperm can survive for up to five or even seven days in the body. Sperm can also make the journey up to the fallopian tube even when ejaculation was outside the vagina.

Methods of contraception basically rely on either:

- Preventing the production of a viable egg.
- Preventing the implantation of an egg once it has been fertilized.
- Putting a barrier between egg and sperm and so preventing their meeting.

- Killing sperm before it can get to the egg.
- A combination of some of these methods.

In trying to make up your mind about a method of contraception, you need to apply exactly the same decision-making techniques we discussed in the previous chapter. You need information, a willingness to discuss your options and feelings, and time to do all this. Again, leaflets and information are available from a variety of sources listed on page 95. Both friends and professional helpers can be useful to you. Your own doctor may be your first port of call.

However, some methods are not available from your family doctor. Condoms, for instance, can only be prescribed on the NHS by clinics or bought in shops. Many doctors do not have the appropriate training or the practice necessary for them to fit an IUD. Some family doctors will prefer to prescribe the Pill rather than other methods, because doing so is quicker and easier than other methods. When a patient has had difficulties in using some methods and is clearly unhappy with what is on offer, quite a few doctors may not be able or willing to spend the time to discuss *why* this is happening. They may instead be tempted to pass the buck and end their involvement by suggesting sterilization. The doctors may not even realize this is what they are doing, but explain their bias in terms of its being the 'best' choice for you. What may get overlooked is how you *feel* about this choice, and how it effects your later actions.

Having explored what we want from a method of contraception and made ourselves aware of how our partners and medical advisers may feel, the next stage is to become familiar with all the methods. To make a free choice, you need to know what *is* available and how to use it.

Contraceptive methods

There are five non-permanent methods that, like sterilization, are totally separated from the actual act of love and are extremely effective. These are the four hormonal methods (oral contraception, injectable contraception, implants and vaginal ring) and the IUD.

Oral contraception

Oral contraception, comes in two basic types – combined and progestogen-only.

Combined oral contraception

These are pills which consist of a measured daily dose of two hormones – synthetic forms of oestrogen and progesterone. They work by affecting the hypothalamus and the pituitary gland. The hormones that trigger ovulation are suppressed and, as long as these pills are taken regularly, egg cells do not ripen in the ovaries and so pregnancy cannot occur.

In the early days of the Pill, quite a high dose of oestrogen was used. Later studies proved that this was associated with health risks and side effects. Recent new advances have resulted in very low dose pills being made available. These suit most women and reduce side effects while still offering complete contraceptive protection.

The most widely used combined pills are presented in packages of 21 pills. You take one a day for three weeks, have seven days free of pill taking and then resume the daily regimen. During the seven days off the Pill, you will experience menstrual bleeding. Although the package is marked to show the day or number in the cycle of each pill to aid your memory, each tablet contains the same formula. However, there are combined pills called biphasic or triphasic (two-or three-step) which vary their strength through the cycle. While it would not matter if you got out of sequence on the ordinary combined pill, biphasic or triphasic pills *must* be taken in the correct order. By giving you a different content of hormones throughout the three weeks of pill-taking, biphasic and triphasic pills are designed to give you a total lower dose of hormones each month. If you find taking a seven-day break upsets the routine of your pill-taking, there are also combined pills that come in packets of 28 with seven of these being inactive sugar pills. Needless to say, these also have to be taken in the right order.

Some women use the Pill to reduce the number of periods they have each year. You can, for instance, take four packets end-to-end, having one week off at the end of a twelve-week period of continuous pill-taking. This would mean you would only have four periods a year. This is actually a healthier and more 'normal' state than having a period each month. A woman's body is designed by nature to be pregnant a large part of its life, not to have thirteen periods a year.

Women who suffer from anaemia might benefit from this regimen. You cannot, however, practise this effect if you are on the bi- or triphasic pill. If you want to miss a period for a special event –

such as a wedding or a holiday – you can safely do this on your own if you are on the conventional combined pill. Just miss out the seven pill-free days by going from one packet straight on to the next and continue taking that until the end of the 21 days. If you are on a bi- or triphasic pill, you can see your doctor or clinic about changing pills for the necessary time. Make sure you go at least a month in advance.

The combined pill, whatever its composition, is virtually 100 per cent effective if taken properly. Pregnancies do sometimes occur for several reasons. Some prescribed or over-the-counter drugs affect digestion and metabolism so that the pill is not absorbed properly and cannot work. Antibiotics such as ampicillin, tetracyclines and rifampicin, most anti-epileptic drugs, some drugs for fungal skin diseases and some tranquillizers, hypnotics, diuretics and analgesics all react in such a way as to prevent the Pill giving you protection. If you lose a pill before it is absorbed, through diarrhoea or vomiting, this too can lead to pregnancy. The worst pills to lose or forget are those at the beginning or the end of a packet. Missing one altogether or taking the last pill early and the first one of a new packet late may well put you at risk. If more than 36 hours passes between one pill and the next, you may be at risk of pregnancy and you should use another method in addition for the next seven days.

Some women on the combined Pill experience side effects such as depression, headaches, nausea, breast tenderness, weight increase, tiredness or a lack of sexual interest. If you do experience these, they are likely to settle down after the first few months of pill-taking. If you wear contact lenses, you might find being on the Pill can be painful as it can make your eyes slightly dry. The combined Pill also could increase your risk of experiencing certain conditions such as thrombosis, high blood pressure and strokes. For this reason, a doctor would need to check your general health – weight, blood pressure and other indications – and to ask about your and your family's health before prescribing you the Pill. Any woman who already has some risk factors such as having blood relatives with such conditions, or who is overweight or smokes, may find her doctor unwilling to prescribe this method of contraception. Women over the age of 30 may also find their doctors increasingly reluctant to prescribe the Pill and many will refuse outright to give the Pill to a woman over 35. However, the latest research does show that as long as none of the other risk factors apply, there is no real reason for a woman having to come off today's low-dose Pills. A healthy women can continue to take the combined contraceptive Pill until menopause.

The main advantage of the combined Pill is that it is so easy. Once part of a routine, pill-taking can be convenient and uncomplicated, and your contraceptive measures need never interrupt or interfere with your lovemaking, however spontaneous and unexpected that might be. The combined Pill has some unexpected medical benefits in that it appears to protect you against cancer of the ovaries and womb, endometriosis, benign breast tumours, pelvic inflammatory disease and possibly rheumatoid arthritis. It can also reduce anaemia, pre-menstrual syndrome and painful or heavy periods. If these problems were a factor in your choosing the Pill and you are now considering sterilization, remember that they may return and perhaps even be worse.

Progestogen-only Pill

Most of the medically dangerous risks associated with the combined Pill are due to its oestrogen content. Women who cannot take this or have been advised to come off it but do want the special convenience of an oral contraceptive may consider the progestogen-only Pill. The progestogen-only Pill is slightly less effective than the combined Pill, with a failure rate of one to four women per 100 over a year. The progestogen-only Pill will stop you ovulating in four out of every ten months. However, this Pill mainly works by thickening the mucus in the cervix, forming a barrier to sperm. It also acts on the endometrium or lining of the womb, so that it rejects any fertilized egg that tries to embed there.

Side effects may include weight gain, headaches, tender breasts or loss of sexual interest, but as with the combined Pill these usually settle down after the first few months of pill-taking. The main difference with the progestogen-only Pill is that the contraceptive effect of this method passes from your body far more quickly than with the combined Pill. You can have up to twelve hours leeway on taking the combined Pill, but if you are more than three hours late taking your progestogen-only Pill, you are at risk. Progestogen-only Pills are packaged in groups of 28 or 35 and are meant to be taken continuously, even through your monthly bleed.

Periods do come every 28 days or so, but can be erratic and some women find they stop altogether. This may be alarming at first since you are unsure whether this is a side effect of the method or if it means that you are pregnant. A total absence of periods usually

33

suggests that ovulation has stopped. One unfortunate risk that the progestogen-only Pill does seem to increase is that of developing an ectopic pregnancy – a pregnancy outside the womb, usually in the fallopian tubes. If you use this method and there is any pain in the lower belly, especially if you have missed or had a delayed or light period, you should see a doctor at once.

Oral contraceptives can only be obtained on prescription and in person from a doctor. However, you can choose whether you see your own family doctor, a doctor at a family planning clinic or indeed any other doctor offering contraceptive advice. This will all be in confidence and totally free on the NHS.

The injectable contraceptive

The 'jab' is an injection of progestogen that works in much the same way as the progestogen-only Pill. It does, however, affect ovulation and so is more effective. The injection is given into the buttock or sometimes into the shoulder muscle. It should be given within five days of your starting a period, and it lasts for eight or twelve weeks at a time, depending on which type you are given. As with the progestogen-only Pill, your periods may become erratic or stop altogether while using this method. Its big advantage is its ease. Apart from a visit to a doctor every two or three months, the user need do nothing and remember nothing else. However, if you *do* experience side effects, such as weight gain, headaches, nausea or depression, these may continue until the effect of the injection wears off. Also, while your fertility will return to normal fairly quickly after using most other methods, delays of up to eighteen months are fairly common after using the injectable contraceptive.

Injectables have generally been used by women in particular circumstances, such as those waiting for a husband's vasectomy to take effect or women who have had a rubella immunization and so must not become pregnant. It is also a first-rate choice for women who find pill-taking routine difficult to keep to, but who need reliable contraception and find other methods unacceptable.

This can include women who have jobs that require they work variable shifts, or women whose home life is erratic. The jab has been the focus of worry and anger from women who feel that it has been used without their consent on those labelled as 'inadequate' by their medical advisers. Whether this is true or not, the method remains the *chosen* contraceptive of many. Any doctor can offer it, free on the NHS.

Implants

Implants are thin, flexible rods about 3.5 cm long, made of plastic and containing progestogen. Six rods are inserted in a fan shape, just under the skin, usually on the arm. They release a steady amount of progestogen which works in the same way as injectable contraception. Implants are possibly the most effective reversible method of contraception. As few as five women in a thousand may get pregnant using implants over a year. Once in place, an implant can be an effetive method of contraception for up to five years. However, if you wanted to get pregnant, you could have them removed and the contraceptive effect stops immediately. Two drawbacks to this method would be that the rods are fairly visible, and that a doctor would need special training to be able to offer this method. You may have to see a hospital doctor to get an implant.

Vaginal rings

The vaginal ring is a soft plastic ring containing progestogen. It is inserted into the vagina where it releases progestogen. The ring is designed to be left in place all the time and will be effective for three months. After this time it will be removed and replaced with another one. The contraceptive vaginal ring works in the same way as the progestogen-only Pill and has a similar effectiveness – around two to three women in every hundred may fall pregnant using it over a year. Vaginal rings are prescribed free on the National Health through any doctor offering contraceptive advice.

Interuterine device (IUD)

Interuterine devices, or IUDs, are small devices made of plastic and copper that fit inside the uterus. It is thought that the presence of a foreign body in the womb encourages a change in secretion. Inflammatory cells and hormones are produced that discourage the egg and sperm from meeting, and fertilized eggs from implanting in the endometrium or lining of the womb. The copper used in IUDs increases this effect and also acts as a sperm-killing substance. The fallopian tubes also react, moving the egg down at a rate which is too quick for fertilization to take place.

The IUD has to be put in place by a trained and experienced doctor or nurse. This is best done towards the end of your period. At this time, the neck of the womb or cervix is softened and the channel through it slightly open.

You may possibly be offered a sedative to help you relax during the procedure and the doctor may inject a small amount of local anaesthetic into the cervix. After checking the size of the uterus, the IUD is passed into the uterus via the vagina. To do this, the doctor uses an 'introducer' – a hollow rod – to deliver the device the right distance inside the body.

After passing the device to the right position inside the uterus, the introducer is removed, leaving the IUD open and in place. Threads attached to the end will trail out of the cervix and these are trimmed to about one to two centimetres long. All you need do in future is to check with an index finger after your period that the threads are still in place, and to have the device changed every three to five years.

IUDs may cause your periods to become longer and heavier, but this is less likely with today's smaller IUDs. Heavier periods from IUD use may be your reason for thinking about changing to sterilization. If so, you would be strongly advised to consider and explore the situation first. It would be a good idea to change to a barrier method for a time and see what happens. You might find that your periods have become longer and heavier because of other factors as well, such as age, and that removing the IUD would not make a difference. Also, you might find that sterilization itself increases your risks of having heavy periods.

IUDs may also be associated with infection that might result in pelvic inflammatory disease (PID). Women who are not in mutually faithful, stable relationships are not advised to use the IUD. For this reason, young women who have not settled down or completed their families and who could thus be more likely to change their partners more often, may find their doctor advising against IUD use. Some women find having an IUD fitted an uncomfortable procedure. This can be helped by seeing the IUD first and seeing how small it is. Sometimes the IUD comes out (expulsion). The device may also be expelled through the uterine wall into the pelvic cavity. This is called a perforation. Perforations, however, are rare (fewer than one in a thousand women) and are mostly likely to happen when the device is put in by an inexperienced doctor. This is why it is really important to see a doctor who fits these devices regularly and who has been properly trained to do so. The IUD shares with the progestogen-only Pill an increased risk of ectopic pregnancy. It is, however, a very reliable method. Some 97–99 per cent of women using it over a year find it protects them from a pregnancy. IUDs are available free from family doctors and family planning clinics.

Barrier contraception

There are five methods that work by preventing the meeting of sperm and egg. They are the barrier methods of male condom, female condom, diaphragm or cap, sponge and spermicide.

The male condom

The male condom or sheath is a thin rubber tube designed to cover the penis during lovemaking and to contain the man's semen after climax. The male condom can be put on by the man or his partner, or they can do it together. Male condoms come packed in threes or dozens, and each individual male condom is sealed in its own foil or plastic wrapper. Male condoms come rolled up, and the idea is that you place one on the end of the erect penis and unroll the device down the length of the penis, like putting on a rolled-up stocking.

If you are to use a male condom successfully and happily there are some important points to note. If you start making love first and then withdraw to put on the male condom, you may risk pregnancy. The male condom must be put on *before* having genital-to-genital contact. Male condoms can leak or even burst if you don't leave a space at the sealed end to take the man's sperm when he comes. So, as you place it on the erect penis, pinch the end of the male condom to leave a loose catchment area. Male condoms can also leak or burst if they are even slightly damaged while being put on. Make sure ragged fingernails, rings or the edge of the packaging do not snag the device as you handle it.

Another threat to the sheath is the use of any oil-based product such as vaseline or baby oil. Both can perish the rubber in a surprisingly short time. If you want to use a lubricating product to aid or add extra fun to lovemaking, use the special jellies such as KY or Durex Lubricating Jelly for vaginal use, and a non-oil massage or moisturizing cream for the rest of your body. Male condoms can slip off and spill semen inside the woman if the man relaxes and remains inside her after he climaxes. It is a good idea for him to withdraw fairly soon after having his orgasm, using one or two fingers firmly to hold the male condom in place as he does so – or for the woman to do it for him. Male condoms are designed for one use only – it is a false economy and very unwise to wash and re-use them. You are also strongly advised to look for the British Standard Kite mark on the package and to buy only approved brands. Using two male condoms at once does *not* improve their efficiency but makes them even more likely to rub two layers against each other and burst. If you want to be particularly reassured, there are 'stronger' varieties on sale.

Male condoms do suffer from an image problem. They have been used for centuries as a protection from sexually transmitted diseases as well as pregnancy, and many of us still associate them with disease and illicit sex. Men and women can be put off buying supplies for fear of the reactions of the person behind the counter or their sexual partner. Men can be particularly frightened of using one in case their awkward fumbling suggests inexperience. Men might also refuse to use a male condom on the grounds that it spoils their pleasure – a claim very much out of date with new materials that can be made into an extraordinarily thin product. In reality, their dread is often that they might lose an erection while trying to put the male condom on, or trigger a premature ejaculation.

On the plus side, male condoms are an extremely effective method of birth control if used with care. According to some studies, as few as two women in a hundred will become pregnant over a year's continuous use. Other studies show higher failure rates, but this is clearly linked to the commitment or expertise of the users, rather than a failure of the method itself. You can increase the effectiveness of the male condom by using spermicides and many sheaths now have their own spermicidal lubrication.

Male condoms are also a valuable protection against many sexually transmitted diseases. By preventing the exchange of body fluids, male condoms are likely to give some protection against HIV, the virus that can cause AIDS. Also, since cervical infection, in young women particularly, is associated with an increased risk of developing pre-cancerous cell changes, barrier contraception may protect against cancer of the cervix.

Male condoms can be very useful in other ways. If you and your partner are spontaneous lovers and like to have intercourse in the morning or just before going out, or even in the open air, you will know how annoying it can be to seep semen afterwards. Doctors and sexual experts are fond of labelling any woman who finds this inconvenient as being a compulsive neurotic with an obsession about hygiene. Such an 'expert' has obviously never had to laugh off a tell-tale damp patch.

Male condoms are available, free, to both men and women from family planning clinics although they are not available from general practitioners. They are also now on sale at pharmacies, supermarkets and some cosmetic and fashion stores. They have no health risks or side effects apart from the occasional allergy or reaction to rubber or the chemicals used in the lubrication and spermicide. Allergy sheaths with hypoallergenic lubrication are available in such a situation.

The female condom

The female condom combines features of both the male condom and the diaphragm and is intended as a protection against sexually transmitted diseases as well as pregnancy. The device is a loose-fitting, soft polyurethane sheath designed to line the vagina. The open end is attached to a flexible ring which lies against the vulva. A separate ring can be dropped into the closed end of the sheath and this is used just like a diaphragm to guide the liner inside the vagina. Once in, the ring anchors the female condom by lodging around the cervix. Alternatively, the female condom can be inserted in the same way as a male condom, by being placed over the penis before penetration.

There are several advantages to the female condom over the male condom. One is that it can be inserted before the man is erect and, since it stays in place whether he is erect or not, the couple can lie together after making love. Couples report less loss of sensation than a male condom because of its loose fit. It will not be damaged by oil or oil-based creams. The main advantage of this method is that it provides an extremely good measure of protection against the spread of disease since both the vagina and much of the vulva are covered by a non-permeable barrier. Since the female condom is under the woman's control, this would allow the female partner to insist on a barrier method being used, even when her partner believes 'It's like taking a shower with your wellies on'. The female condom is available from some family planning clinics and from pharmacies.

Diaphragm and cap

The names diaphragm and cap tend to be used as interchangeable but in fact they describe two slightly different variations on the same method. Both are devices which are made of rubber that are placed in the vagina to form a barrier preventing the passage of sperm into the uterus. The diaphragm is the more popular of the two. It is a dome of rubber with a rim that contains a coil or strip of metal to make it pliable yet firm. Diaphragms can be from 55 mm to 100 mm in diameter. They are designed to lie at a slant across the upper end of the vagina. In this position, a correctly fitted diaphragm will be held in place and will not be dislodged by lovemaking. However, since the inner third of the vagina does enlarge during sexual excitement, the device probably does not provide a consistent barrier. For this reason, you are advised always to use a sperm-killing cream or jelly in addition. Indeed, diaphragms are often considered to be no more than a way of carrying spermicide to the cervix and holding it there.

A diaphragm is inserted by the woman, or her partner, at any time prior to making love. If this is done within three hours of lovemaking, spermicidal cream or jelly is spread on the rubber dome which is then squeezed and folded to make it tampon-shaped and sized. This is guided into the vagina and pushed up until it unfolds at the top of the vault, covering the cervix. With the middle or index finger, the user checks that the cervix can be felt through the rubber of the dome, and thus that the device is in place over it. If the diaphragm is put in more than three hours ahead of intercourse, spermicide can be left off and added nearer the time of lovemaking.

Caps are smaller in size and are designed to fit closely over the cervix itself. They stay there by suction and are close-fitting enough not to need spermicides.

Both diaphragms and caps must be left in place for at least six hours after having sex, to give any spermicide a chance to work and to allow normal acidity in the vagina also to kill sperm. If you make love a second or even third time, you are advised to top up your spermicide and to count the six hours before removing your device from the last act of intercourse. To remove a cap you need to knock the device off the cervix with a fingertip before hooking it out. A diaphragm is drawn out with one or two fingers. Women with short fingers or long vaginas can use a special remover to do this.

After use, the diaphragm or cap is washed in warm water. Before storing it in its own container, hold the device up to the light and check for holes or cracks.

Women are often put off trying a diaphragm or cap by people who describe this method as messy or inconvenient. In fact, it is no more messy than lovemaking itself, hardly a dry, dignified event if done with enjoyment. It is no more inconvenient to put in a diaphragm or cap than it is to take off your clothes before making love. Used consistently, these two methods have a very low failure rate – as few as two women in a hundred using such a device for a year might become pregnant. Female barrier methods also offer some protection against cervical and pelvic infections and against cancer of the cervix.

The disadvantages are that you *do* need to plan ahead or to be confident enough to call a halt during foreplay, either to put in the device or the spermicide. If you use this method you should also be happy about handling yourself intimately, and to find it easy to do so. Women with disabilities or from cultures that allow them to touch their genitals with only one hand may find this difficult, or need a partner's co-operation. Diaphragms also have one disadvantage in that they may increase your chance of developing cystitis. This is because the rim can be pressed against delicate tissue by your partner's movements and set up inflammation. If this happens, checking the fit of your diaphragm or changing to a cervical cap should solve the problem. Some men find they can feel the device in place, and women can experience a certain loss of sensation. Although the cervix and vaginal vault are not particularly rich in nerve endings, many women can feel the man ejaculating and this may trigger their own orgasms.

The muscle tone of the vagina can change over a period of time. Age, or trauma due to a birth, miscarriage or abortion, or a loss or gain of weight of more than three kilograms or half a stone can make a diaphragm or cap that did fit suddenly ineffective. After any such change, or every six to twelve months, this should be checked by a doctor or nurse. Since a good fit *is* so important, and can best be worked out by a trained professional, you must get your vaginal barrier method from a doctor or nurse to begin with. If you lose or damage your device and have no reason to feel any change has taken place, you can replace it over-the-counter from a chemist. They are free, however, from family doctors and clinics, with a regular supply of spermicides.

The sponge

A relatively new variation on a very old theme is the contraceptive sponge. This is a disposable device made of polyurethane foam. Natural sponges soaked in vinegar or lemon juice have been used as birth control devices for centuries, but the modern sponge improves on this idea. It is impregnated with a spermicide and is very absorbent. The device is around 5.5 cm in diameter and some 2.5 cm thick. On one side there is a deep dimple, and a loop of material is attached. To use it, you moisten the sponge to activate the spermicide and push it high into your vagina until the dimple rests over the cervix. The sponge must be left in place for six hours after lovemaking, but it can be put in as much as 24 hours beforehand and sex can take place at any time and as often as you like during this period. The device is removed by hooking the loop with a finger and pulling it out. It is then thrown away.

The obvious advantages of the sponge are that it is not only free of mess in itself but also soaks up semen. It can be inserted quite some time before lovemaking and no extra precautions then need to be remembered. Like a condom, it can be bought from virtually any pharmacy at a moment's notice. It is also available free from some family planning clinics. There are no side effects or health risks. The major disadvantage is that it has a high failure rate of 9 to 25 per cent.

Spermicides

Spermicides are chemicals that form a barrier to stop and destroy sperm. They come in the form of creams or jellies, aerosol foams, pessaries or film. Creams or jellies may be squeezed from their tubes onto diaphragms and caps. They can also be put into an applicator – a syringe with a blunt nozzle – that is then inserted into the vagina and the contents pushed out into the vagina. Aerosol foams are used in this way as well. Pessaries are a solid gel made in a tampon-like shape, which are pushed up into the vagina and left for a few minutes to melt. The solid film can be inserted into the vagina with a finger or draped over a diaphragm.

Spermicides not only act on sperm, but also on germs. There is ample evidence that a wide range of sexually transmitted diseases, including HIV, the virus that can lead to AIDS, are inactivated by the chemical Nonoxynol-9, which is a major ingredient in most spermicides today. Spermicides also form a barrier protecting against the risk of cancer of the cervix.

Spermicides seem to have a poor record for contraceptive efficiency on their own, although studies disagree on this. An American study, for instance, showed that a large group of well motivated women had as few as four pregnancies per hundred over a year's use – as good as the IUD, diaphragm or condom. Other studies suggest a lower efficiency, probably on a par with the sponge. Spermicides improve the efficiency of other barrier methods and on their own are certainly better than nothing. They are also effective in cases where you already have a reduced risk of becoming pregnant, such as when fertility wanes approaching and during the menopause.

Spermicides carry no health risks, although a few women or their partners may experience a reaction to the chemicals used. Doctors and clinics can prescribe them free, or they can be bought over-the-counter without the need for a visit to a doctor or other health professional.

Other contraceptive methods

There are two methods of contraception that may become both more acceptable and safer as you grow older and less fertile.

Fertility awareness

This is also known as periodic abstinence or natural family planning (NFP), although it may also be known by the old terms Rhythm Method or Safe Period. It works by avoiding sex at the times in your menstrual cycle when you are most likely to conceive, that is, around ovulation. Couples can use a variety of techniques to find out the female partner's fertile times and abstain for several days before and after this occurs.

There are three basic ways of finding out when ovulation is likely to occur: the calendar method; the temperature method and the cervical mucus or Billings method.

The calendar method In the calendar method, you keep a record of your periods over a time and use that information to predict the probable 'safe' days. Such predictions are unlikely to be exact. Even women who think they have a regular cycle will find that each month is slightly different. Women's menstrual cycles vary from anything between 21 to 42 days between periods. This makes anticipating the next ovulation a bit difficult. The day on which you release an egg is not affected by when you had your *last* bleed. It is, however, linked to when you have your *next* period. This is because ovulation is part of the process that leads up to this event. Ovulation is almost always followed by a period fourteen days later. However, it is not uncommon for periods to arrive twelve to sixteen days after ovulation.

If you keep a record of the first day of your period for at least six, and preferably twelve, months, you can work out the likely spread of the safe and unsafe days in following months. You do this by taking the *shortest* cycle, say 26 days, and subtracting from it the figure eighteen. In this case, that gives you eight. You then take the longest cycle, say 35 days, and take from it the figure ten. In this case, you are left with 25. This would mean that your first unsafe day in any cycle is likely to be eight days after the beginning of your period, and your last unsafe day is likely to be 25 days after the beginning of your last period. To be safe from pregnancy using these calculations would mean that you could only make love up until the seventh day after the period starts, and on the 26th day onwards. Of course, in a 26-day cycle in which your bleeding lasts for seven days, this would allow you only two days of safe sex, unless you and your partner have no objection to having intercourse during menstruation. In a particularly short cycle, however, this in itself could be risky, as sperm may then survive long enough to be waiting for the next ovulation. This method is no longer recommended to be used on its own.

The temperature method Just after ovulation your temperature drops very slightly and then rises until a few days before your next period. You can see this dip and peak if you take and note down your temperature each morning *before* getting up or doing anything to raise it (such as having a hot drink).

After three consecutive days at the raised temperature, you will be safe to have sex. Ovulation will have occurred and by this time the egg will have decayed to a point where it is unlikely to be fertilized. If you keep a regular chart and your cycle is extremely stable, you may well feel confident enough to work out which days in the cycle are safe *before* ovulation is likely to happen. However, since sperm can survive for as long as five to seven days, and even in the most regular cycle ovulation can happen earlier than you expect, you may only be able to allow yourself between one and four days after your period has stopped. Strictly speaking, the only time that you can be really sure it is 'safe' using this method is *after* ovulation. In a regular 28-day cycle, this would amount to around ten days each month.

If you want to pursue this method, you would be advised to discuss it with your own doctor or one at a family planning clinic, or through a trained ovulation method teacher (see Useful Addresses). You would also be advised to use the special, free thermometer and charts they can give you. Your temperature can be raised by illness and lowered by medicines such as aspirin – so you should be on the lookout for inaccurate readings.

The cervical mucus or Billings method Unlike the temperature method, successful use of the cervical mucus method gives you some early-warning signal of the approach of ovulation. Three to four days before an egg is released, your body begins to ready itself for conception. The cervix releases a flow of mucus which mingles with the regular flow of liquid from the walls of the vagina. Throughout most of the cycle the cervical and vaginal secretions are cloudy and somewhat thick. This is infertile mucus. Around the time of ovulation, the cervix produces 'fertile mucus' which is quite different from infertile mucus in that it feels wetter and is clear, stretchy and thin. This fertile cervical mucus is designed to help sperm on its way through the cervical canal and on up the womb into the fallopian tubes.

Users of this method should avoid intercourse from as soon as they notice an increase in vaginal wetness until they have been relatively dry again for four days. A further test to check whether you are producing fertile mucus is to rub a small amount between two fingers and then separate them. If the mucus is slippery and elastic in texture, and stretches for a few centimetres before breaking, it is likely to be pre-ovulatory cervical mucus. However, if your cycle is short, you may find that the warning change happens during or just after your period and so can be missed.

Combinations of methods The most effective option is to combine several of these methods, taking your temperature but also watching for changes in mucus and other signs such as *mittle-schmertz* to indicate ovulation is about to happen or has happened. *Mittleschmertz*, or 'middle pain', is a gripping pain experienced by many women in the lower belly at the time of ovulation.

Using a combination of ways of detecting ovulation is called the sympto-thermal method. If you have had the opportunity of learning from a good teacher and use natural family planning with care, fertility awareness can be as much as 80 to 98 per cent effective. That is, used by 100 women over a year, between two and twenty women will become pregnant using them.

As the term 'periodic abstinence' suggests, the point of all these elaborate charts and observations is to find out the most likely time of the month for conception and to avoid having sex on these days. Enthusiastic users of the method claim several advantages for it. There are no physical side effects or health risks and the method is accepted by religions and cultures that otherwise frown on birth control. The method is under the couple's personal control, and once established is always available – even when pharmacies and doctors' surgeries are closed. The communication and closeness necessary to make such a method work are said to bring a couple together, and restricting sex to certain days gives it the spice of anticipation.

Natural family planning can be particularly successful for the confident and stable couple who can make what would be an inconvenience for people not in a stable relationship a plus in their own.

Temperature charts, special thermometers and training on using all these ways of calculating your ovulation are available from your own family doctor or practice nurse, a nurse or doctor at a family planning clinic, or from the Natural Family Planning Service.

Other ways of finding out when you are fertile You can now buy special kits from a chemist that show when ovulation is due. These work on the fact that one or two days before ovulation takes place, your body increases production of a hormone called Luteinizing Hormone (LH). This can be found in your urine and by testing with a special sampler you can have warning of the approach of ovulation. The drawback is that you only have one or two days notice, so intercourse immediately before a positive test is very likely to make you pregnant. The kits are actually intended for use by couples who are planning a pregnancy and as such give an excellent indication of when to make love to increase your chances of starting a baby. They could, however, be a valuable addition in giving a clear signal for when ovulation has happened, allowing you to be sure you are safe for the rest of the month. However, at the moment, the kits are an extremely expensive aid to natural methods of contraception.

Coitus interruptus

Another method that is usually criticized as being unsafe but that might merit a second look as you get older is coitus interruptus, also known as withdrawal, 'pulling out' or 'being careful'. In this, the man withdraws his penis before ejaculation and 'comes', or has his orgasm, outside his partner. The theory is that if semen is not deposited inside the woman there is no risk of pregnancy. It is probably the oldest method of birth control, apart from infanticide and abortion.

Coitus interruptus has a bad reputation and the main disadvantage is said to be its inefficiency. Living sperm can be found in the lubricating fluid that oozes from the penis *before* ejaculation. By the time the man withdraws, sperm may already be on its way towards a meeting with the ovum. However, various studies of the method do not appear to bear this out. Among highly motivated couples, the failure rate from withdrawal can be the same as the failure rate from mechanical means of contraception, such as diaphragms. As with most methods, the key seems to be whether or not the users are happy to employ it and are confident and practised.

The advantages of withdrawal are that it requires no preparation at all – no charts, no pills, no bits and pieces. It cannot be lost, forgotten when you go away, or left off the shopping list. It has no physical side effects. Its critics claim that, just as with periodic abstinence, the method causes stress. Pulling out makes the experience incomplete for the man and unsatisfactory for the woman. Furthermore, fear of pregnancy means that the woman is unable to relax and enjoy lovemaking.

All of this may be true when the method is used hastily by an inexperienced couple. Its failures are a result of a general lack of experience and communication. *If* the couple agree that this is to be their chosen method, practise its use so that the man *does* pull out in time and make sure that the female partner is sexually satisfied, there is no reason why the method need not be satisfactory. Methods which affect lovemaking itself, either by barring it at certain times or interrupting it each time, are acceptable to some people all the time or to most of us at some time.

Our reservations about these methods are often based on a rather unyielding attitude to what we see as the 'right' way to make love. Up to now, the understanding has been that sexual expression consists of a man and a woman caressing each other as a prelude to 'the real thing' – the insertion of penis into vagina. Once in, thrusting movements result in a satisfying and preferably simultaneous climax for both partners, which ends the encounter.

In practice, most couples have always made variations on this theme – involving oral sex, mutual masturbation and, in some cases, anal penetration. The majority of women do not have an orgasm from straight, man-on-top penetrative sex but find that clitoral stimulation from hands, lips or tongue, or from the woman-on-top position, is needed for full mutual enjoyment. Fear of HIV/AIDS has meant that many people have changed their attitudes to what is normal or desirable sexual practice. The necessary medical advice that exchange of body fluids should be avoided has led many couples to find that penetrative sex is not the be-all-and-end-all of sex. By giving each other pleasure by using other parts of their bodies except genital-to-genital exchanges, many couples have found that avoiding putting semen inside the woman need not be a chore, but can be a natural part of even more exciting sex than intercourse. For this reason, withdrawal as a method of birth control may soon be seen in a more positive light.

Which method?

In choosing a method, you need to know not which is the 'best' method, but to work out which one suits *you*. You and your partner need to find out what it is you want most from your contraception. Is it absolute protection from pregnancy? Total freedom to be spontaneous? A measure of protection from various forms of cancer or sexually transmitted disease? An absence of side effects or health risks? Freedom from a flow of vaginal secretions afterwards? To use a method efficiently, you need to be comfortable, and any distaste or lingering fears about the choice you have made, or which has been made for you, is likely to have an unsatisfactory outcome.

Having made a choice, it is also important to note that you and your circumstances may well change. That being so, what was right for one time may no longer be right for you now. There are times in your life when it may be most important to be free from the fear of pregnancy. There are times when you are dithering over the decision to become pregnant and might welcome the opportunity to let chance or nature take a hand. As you age, methods that might have been unacceptable due to lack of confidence or embarrassment become easy. Methods that might have been risky become safer as your fertility declines.

Most couples may find a typical contraceptive life history goes as follows. They could use a condom at first, for protection against sexual infection and cancer as well as pregnancy. Then, they may move on to the Pill for a few years until their first child, using the cap just before a planned pregnancy and the IUD in the intervals between children. After probable completion of family, they may mix diaphragm or cap, condom and sponge use for a few years before deciding on sterilization. They may keep a supply of condoms and sponges as a back-up in case any of their other methods fail.

Even if you think that you and your partner have been through these methods and found them lacking, think one more time before rejecting them all. A method you found unpleasant years ago, or that a doctor suggested was not suitable, may now be more acceptable or appropriate. Before taking the final irrevocable step to be sterilized, cast your mind over the rest. If, having given them a fair hearing, you still decide they are no longer for you, you are genuinely ready to go about arranging your sterilization.

Case histories

Gordon's and Mary's story

Mary had been using an IUD for several years after the birth of her second child. Both she and Gordon were happy with their family and sure that a boy and a girl were enough. When she began to have heavy and uncomfortable periods, a friend suggested that she ask her doctor about being sterilized. 'We talked it over and I was quite keen; it did seem a good solution and I was always a bit nervous about the coil. A friend of mine had an ectopic pregnancy with one, and I wasn't a 100 per cent sure it was working. You do like to be certain about your birth control, don't you?'

Gordon, however, was not keen on the idea. He found it difficult to explain why. The two of them saw their family doctor, who made time for them outside ordinary surgery hours to discuss the matter without pressure. He helped Gordon to put his feelings into words. While Mary would have been happy to be sterilized, it became clear that for Gordon a certain something might be missing if either of them had this operation at this time. The doctor also warned that, although the IUD might be the culprit in making Mary's periods uncomfortable, it could also be due to her age – late thirties – and that female sterilization itself could also have this effect. He discussed other methods of birth control with them. Both partners had dismissed the idea of barrier methods out of hand as being 'bothersome and messy', and were surprised when their doctor urged them to give it a try.

'It then struck us that Mary had never used a diaphragm and that my only experience of condoms was as a clumsy and very nervous teenager. We did try them and were pleasantly surprised. Even collapsing in hysterical giggles when trying to put on a coloured sheath didn't spoil it – it made lovemaking fun. I mean, who says you shouldn't laugh while you're making love to your wife?' Gordon and Mary decided to try sheaths and a diaphragm, using them turn and turn about. Once Mary had been reassured that she was less fertile and thus less likely to fall pregnant than when she had been younger, she felt able to trust these methods. The couple agreed to use barrier methods for a few more years and to defer a decision on sterilization until both felt happy about it.

Robert's and Alice's story

Alice had been on the Pill since she was eighteen and was perfectly happy with this as a method of contraception. So she was particularly upset when her doctor told her that after her next birthday – her 35th – he would not be prepared to prescribe this method any more. He gave her leaflets on barrier methods, the IUD and sterilization, and said she would have to choose between them, but if she was sure her family was complete, he strongly recommended that she was sterilized. Alice was furious. She had always thought that sterilization was a method for 'older women' and didn't exactly feel like putting herself in that category. After talking with several friends of the same age, she went to see a woman doctor who saw patients just for contraceptive advice. 'I must admit it was really in desperation, because I didn't expect her to say anything different. I mean, you think doctors are all going to say the same thing, don't you? Well, she said I could do two things. I could go on a different type of Pill. She said that the progestogen-only Pill would be perfectly safe for me whatever my age, but that it was slightly less effective than the other kind. Or, she said, I could stay on my present Pill but I would have to give up smoking and lose some weight. Well, I had a chat to Robert about this and we both thought that all in all it might not be a bad idea. We've got these friends who live down the road who have taken up jogging and playing squash at our local leisure centre, and you should see the difference it's made to them. Giving up smoking was a real nuisance, but I used the money I saved to buy some gorgeous track suits and in only six months I've lost half a stone. This woman doctor says I can stay on the Pill for as long as I like, as long as I stay fit and healthy, but I think I'll be ready for a sterilization in a few more years.'

3

Where to go to get your operation

We have this really old fashioned GP. He's great when you're ill, especially for the kiddies, but when I asked about a vasectomy I could tell I'd shocked him rigid. Well, we didn't know what to do after that. As far as I was concerned, a private operation would cost a bomb and anyway we had no idea where to go to find out about it.

Stan W

You may have gone through your decision-making on your own or you may have involved your own doctor in your deliberations. Whichever, when it comes to taking the next step – actually putting this in motion and getting the operation done – the best person to see first is your own general practitioner. For many reasons, your own doctor should be aware of what you are planning. If your doctor is sympathetic to your request, he or she is likely to be able to smooth your path and offer you advice and assistance. Very few doctors now have a moral or religious objection to helping their patients to obtain contraceptive help. If yours has reservations about this particular request, it may be worthwhile at least listening to what is being said.

Whatever the attitude to your having this operation, your doctor *needs* to know it has been carried out in order to make proper diagnoses in the future. For instance, he or she may not treat symptoms that suggest pregnancy with an appropriate urgency if it isn't known that you had taken surgical steps to prevent this happening. Your own doctor will be the one on hand if anything goes wrong or you have any worries or questions after the operation, so it is a good idea to keep him or her in the picture. In any case, two of the three routes open to you are best, or in some cases only, started through your own family doctor.

In this country, you can obtain a sterilization operation from three basic sources; the National Health Service, a private surgeon, and through a charity. Your own doctor could save you time and money by sending you to the right place or advising you on what to do.

51

Both male and female sterilizations are available in the UK on the National Health Service. You can't go directly to a hospital for an NHS operation but must be referred by a doctor. To refer you, the doctor sees you first and discusses the matter with you and your partner. When all of you are happy that the right decision has been made, or if your doctor feels that a further talk with a surgeon would help you to make up your mind, an appointment is made for you. The doctor sends a letter of introduction to the hospital surgeon, or gives it to you to take along. The letter may support your request and say why the doctor thinks this is acceptable. Or, it may just explain what you have asked and leave it to the hospital doctor to make up his or her mind. Don't assume that because your doctor does send you on that he or she agrees with what you are doing.

In most cases the referring doctor has to be your own family GP, although under some circumstances a doctor from a family planning clinic might arrange the referral. When you see the hospital doctor, you may be asked to go back over the same ground that you have covered with your own doctor. This is not needless repetition. For a start, you may have changed your mind or at least become less sure in the time between one appointment and the next. Also, your own doctor cannot write down everything you have said and the surgeon needs to discuss your feelings as much as does your own doctor. In fact, he or she has even more right. If you do change your mind after the operation and are upset about it, the surgeon is the person you're likely to blame. To protect themselves, doctors need to be able to state in your medical notes that the operation was fully discussed with you and you agreed to it.

Last but not least, you need the opportunity to talk with the surgeon, or a member of the team, who will be doing your operation, to ask all the questions about the procedure that may be worrying you. At the end of this consultation you may be given a date for your operation, or told that you will be advised. Female sterilizations and vasectomies can be performed in a hospital, with either the man or woman going in for a few hours as a day case or a woman going in overnight as an in-patient.

However, the biggest stumbling block you may encounter in your search for a free sterilization is money. Not *your* money as such, but the funding available and set aside for family planning in your area. Each Health District has a fixed annual budget for its health care. Allocations are made to different departments, one of them being family planning. Most family planning departments then allocate a fixed sum each year to be spent on sterilizations in their hospitals. It may sound odd, but each operation done in a hospital is costed out and the sum marked down to the relevant department. Surgeons and anaesthetists also receive fees from the National Health Service for taking part in what are seen as special, extra procedures over and above their normal workload. These are called 'item of service fees'. Any action to do with family planning comes under this heading.

When the budget for the year is spent, a particular department may then refuse to do any more sterilizing operations until the beginning of a new financial year. Pressure on a department may cause a waiting list of up to nine months – time enough for you to have yet one more addition to your family before getting your operation. Of course, some doctors see sterilization as just part part of their job and refuse to claim the special fees for it, so extending the budget in their hospitals. Some areas have more demand than others, so it is always worth finding out through your own doctor about the situation locally. Remember also that a GP has the right to refer a patient to any hospital in the country. You and your doctor could find out which hospitals have short or no waiting lists and you could be referred there. A GP can also do a vasectomy for free in his or her surgery, and some trained family doctors will do so. The only problem is that providing such a service will actually cost the practice a certain amount of money. Not only is the doctor's time involved, but a nurse may have to be paid to be there. And, of course, the doctor would have to buy surgical gloves, instruments and other articles. However, some do think it worthwhile in patient and job satisfaction. You may be lucky and be able to get your sterilization done for free, with the minimum of waiting.

It is worth noting that as a method of contraception sterilization is very cost-effective. If you are in your thirties and would be fertile for around another fifteen years, it could cost the country from 50 per cent to 300 per cent more to finance a diaphragm, condom or IUD, or to keep you on the Pill, than it would to sterilize or vasectomize you. Add to that the cost of any unwanted pregnancy or an abortion, and it is clearly a nonsense to refuse anyone a sterilization on the grounds of expense. And don't forget that the National Health Service is not doing you a free favour. You have *paid* for this service out of your contributions and taxes.

However, administrators are not always logical and you may find it difficult to get your sterilization in a reasonable time scale. If so, you can obtain a male or a female sterilization by seeing a surgeon privately. The advantage of this, of course, is that you are almost certain to find the waiting period considerably shorter than that for an NHS operation. Most surgeons doing private operations can offer you a date within a few weeks to suit your own timetable. They are also more likely to treat you as a 'client' or 'customer' rather than a 'patient'. You are advised not to take advantage of this relationship. If an NHS surgeon refuses to operate because he or she feels you or your youngest child are too young, your marriage is shaky or your reasons are suspect, you may be tempted to storm off and get what you want by paying for it. However sure you feel at the time, it might be a good idea to listen to the objections and think about them. But if you have been considering sterilization for some time and are sure of your decision, it might seem worth the money not to have to wait around any longer.

Your GP would refer you to a surgeon who does private operations. The advantage of going through your own doctor is that you have a pretty good guarantee of the surgeon's competence. Your doctor will know who does such operations regularly in your area and can recommend the best (although this will not always be the cheapest). The chances are that it will be the surgeon whose waiting lists at your own hospital are so full. Of course, you *can* see a doctor who has a private practice without having to go through your own GP. The drawback is that unless you have a very good reason to know what you are doing you may not choose the best person for the job. You may also find yourself paying over the odds. Unless your own doctor has a particular religious or moral objection against sterilization, go through him or her. Alternatively, your own family doctor may do vasectomies in his or her surgery for a fee. More and more doctors are offering this facility.

Another route you can follow is to go to one of the specialist charities that work in the birth control field. Agencies such as British Pregnancy Advisory Service, Pregnancy Advisory Service, and Marie Stopes House all run clinics that provide female sterilization and/or vasectomies. Their charges are fair and in some cases you may be able to pay over a period of time or even have a reduced fee. Some Health Authorities use these charities as agents, having found it costs less to pay BPAS, PAS or Marie Stopes to do the operations than to have them done on NHS time in NHS premises. Since doctors working for these charities do frequent operations, it can be argued that the service they offer is better and safer than that given in many NHS hospitals. If you want to go to one of the charities, you can do so direct without a referral from your own doctor. You simply ring or write for an appointment.

Charitable agencies will require that you attend a counselling session to discuss your reasons for seeking the operation, as would an NHS surgeon. They are ethically bound to try to ensure you do not make a decision in haste or under pressure that you might regret. The agreed system now is that individuals requesting sterilization should be seen for counselling at an appointment prior to the operation itself. When you go through your own GP, only the person having the operation may be asked to attend this – the understanding being that joint discussions with the couple have already been held. Some NHS doctors and most private surgeons or charities are likely to ask both parties to come along. Some surgeons also ask the partner to sign or at least agree to a consent form. This is a formal document that is completed for all operations. In signing it, you state that you understand what is being done and give your surgeon permission to do the work. Strictly speaking, adults have total rights over their own bodies, and only over their own bodies. Not even a marriage partner can insist on or stop you having an operation. However, with something like sterilization, that affects a marriage and a sexual relationship, any responsible doctor would at least ask that you show good faith by sharing this decision.

Do you have the choice between an NHS or a private operation? The short answer is Yes. Even if money is short, you may be able to pay in instalments, be granted help by a charity, have it paid for by your Health District or even be lent the money by a Bank (they usually enter it under the heading of personal loan rather than house improvements!). So the real question is which route would really suit you best. An NHS operation does not, of course, cost you anything extra on top of your normal NHS contributions. The doctors you will need to see may be helpful, expert and treat you with the utmost care and respect. With a private or charity operation, however, you may find the staff more likely to treat you as a sentient adult, able to have already obtained information and to have made up your mind as a result. Private operations are also far more likely to be conducted in a less formal and more comfortable setting than in a hospital. The private route may be quicker than going through the NHS. However, you could be pleasantly surprised and the best advice is to give your own GP a fair chance before bypassing the usual channels.

Case histories

Jean's and Geoff's story

Jean and Geoff made a joint decision for one of them to be sterilized. When they went to their doctor for her advice and help they had assumed it would be Jean who would have the operation. However, during their discussion, the doctor pointed out that their local hospital had a long waiting list for female sterilizations and wasn't even considering vasectomies at that time. 'Our doctor then said that if we wanted to consider going private, we could have an operation fairly quickly. And that, of course, a vasectomy would be cheaper.'

Since Geoff was just as happy to have the operation as Jean, this made up their minds for them. Says Jean: 'I suppose we're sort of against private medicine in principle, but this just seemed so silly. We weren't happy with our contraception, and here we would have to wait *ages* for a chance to be sterilized and it would virtually *have* to be me having the operation. It would cost the NHS more than giving Geoff the "snip" and it was such a waste. Our doctor recommended a local surgeon who charged us £75 all told. We thought it well worth the money. In fact, it was the sum I'd put aside to buy Geoff a really wonderful 40th birthday present, and he said it was the best birthday present he could have had. He managed to arrange the op for the day of his birthday and I organized a surprise party to welcome him home. He loved it. He sat there with his feet up, holding court and scaring the pants off our friends with lurid descriptions of the operation. They couldn't have been too put off though. Three of them have had the "snip" too since then.'

John's and Sandra's story

John and Sandra had talked about sterilization for over two years before they finally brought up the subject with their family doctor. They had two children, a four-year-old who is theirs and a fourteen-year-old from John's previous marriage. In spite of the fact that both were in their late thirties, they were turned down by their doctor who said that they might want another child of their own. 'I was annoyed,' says Sandra, 'I felt it was a bit of an insult to Andy who I feel *is* my own son. Two are right for us, and it doesn't matter to us who gave birth to them in the first place.

The doctor said it wasn't how *he* felt, but it would be the hospital doctors who would turn us down.'

John wondered if it might be easier to be accepted for sterilization by going private and asked around among friends who had already had the operation. To his surprise, one of them had another suggestion. 'I must admit finances were a bit tight, so even a vasectomy would have been stretching our budget a bit. A friend who lived nearby told me to change doctors and to try his. I didn't know you could do this. The new doctor was far more willing to talk to us and he said that the consultants at the hospital would take each case on its merits and not refuse outright as our old doctor said. Looking back, I don't know whether the old doctor was just out of touch with the hospital doctors or was trying to push his own views but not owning up to it. Anyway, we went to the hospital and they were fine. Sandra went in three months later.'

Six years on, Sandra never regrets her operation. 'I'm glad I had it on the NHS, though,' she says, 'I think you should use the Health service properly. I didn't have any complications, but I was glad my own doctor was there. I'd have felt bad about going to him for any worries over the operation if I'd had it outside the NHS.'

4

The operation

I'm not sure I want to know what they do inside you. No, that's
silly, isn't it? I mean it's your body and you ought to know what
goes on and how it works and what a doctor does to you.

Maureen K

An understanding of exactly *how* a male or female sterilization is
done can help you in making up your mind; either on whether you
will have the operation at all or on which partner will have the
surgery. It is also important to understand that there are more than
just two operations to choose between. Each gender can be
rendered sterile in a variety of ways. Each have their advantages
and disadvantages. While your surgeon may have good reasons for
opting for one particular procedure, you need to know the ins and
outs of these. You may need or want to have some say in which
method is to be used.

When you sign the consent form, either at your initial consultation with the surgeon or when you arrive at the hospital for the
operation, you are likely to find two things. First, the operation you
will be having will be clearly stated. You don't sign up to be
sterilized; you sign up to have a laparoscopic tubal occlusion, or
whatever. This is useful for you. Since you are also supposed to
agree that 'the nature of this operation has been explained to me
and I understand the implications', if it hasn't and as yet you don't,
you have a good excuse to ask for an explanation.

The real reason for specifying the operation is to protect the
surgeon from being sued if you later became pregnant. If the
promise was to sterilize you and it failed, you could sue and win. If
the promise is to occlude or block your tubes, and this *is* done but
fails, you have no come back, since the doctor operated to the best
of ability and in good faith. Of course, if you could prove that the
doctor did not block the tubes properly, you could win a case. The
second thing you will notice is that you are being asked to agree that
you understand that the operation is irrevocable; and that it does
have a risk of failure. You might think these two sit oddly together!
Again, both are points to protect the doctor and are important for
you to note. Sterilization *is* a remarkably effective method of birth

control – but in some unusual cases it does fail. And while reversal operations are available and can work, reversal is not something you should count on.

What happens during female sterilization?

There are over 200 ways of performing a female sterilization, depending on how the surgeon approaches the fallopian tubes and how the tubes are then prevented from delivering an egg to the uterus.

Your surgeon will need to enter your pelvic cavity and he or she can do this through an opening in the abdominal wall or through one at the top of the vagina. Once in, the tubes can be cut, cauterized or have clips or rings put on them to block them.

Early techniques tended to be quite heavy-handed. One surgeon is reported to have sterilized his patients by actually tying their fallopian tubes in a knot – the success of this procedure is not recorded! A Dr Madlener developed a technique that is still known by his name. In the Madlener method, a section of the fallopian tube is crushed by heavy forceps and then tied off. The operation did seem to be effective, but amazingly some women have found that a pregnancy might occur after some years. Another surgeon – Walthardt – went one better by crushing and tying off each tube in two places. But even in some of the cases using his method, pregnancy can still result. The problem is that the human body is astonishingly resiliant. Even a flattened fallopian tube may resurrect itself and once again open a pathway for sperm to reach a fertile egg and the resultant blastocyst to reach the uterus.

Pomeroy was the first surgeon to suggest that a section be cut out of the tubes and the ends tied up to encourage them to seal over and close. Pomeroy's procedure is still used and in some parts of the world is the most common method of female sterilization. However, even here some failures have been recorded. In some cases, the cut ends of the tubes reopen themselves, allowing sperm to make the journey from the uterus up the first section of the tube, across the gap and into the end section, there to meet a waiting egg. Pregnancies have resulted from this. Ectopic pregnancies have also occurred, when the developing egg remains in the tube and attempts to continue its growth there. The fallopian tubes cannot expand to accommodate a pregnancy, and will eventually rupture painfully and sometimes fatally. So, in yet another variation, a Dr

Irving turned the section of the tube still attached to the uterus back on itself. The end is buried in the surface of the uterus and stitched in place to prevent the ends from opening up again.

Today, when you go to the hospital or clinic to have your operation, what is likely to happen to you? You will be asked to report to your hospital or clinic, ready for your operation. If you are having a day care operation, either under general anaesthetic or a local, you will probably be trusted to make some of the important pre-operative checks yourself. If the incision is to be in an area covered by pubic hair, you will be asked to shave. A handy tip here is that hair-removing or depilatory cream is best. You can't cut yourself with cream although you must follow the directions carefully and use the gentler, facial quality. When hair grows back, it is likely to itch less and feel less stubbly than if you use a razor. You will also be asked to arrive fresh from a bath or to have one when you arrive and, if having a general anaesthetic, not to eat for twelve hours beforehand. This last advice is not something to ignore. If you have food in your stomach, you risk vomiting while unconscious. You could choke and die, or inhale and suffocate, or give yourself a nasty case of pneumonia, which also might kill you. So don't be cute about sneaking in a final piece of toast or cup of tea. It could be your last. Some hospitals or clinics prefer to supervise the preparations and have you in the night before your operation.

When everything is ready you will be asked to change into an operating gown – the type that fasten up the back and make you feel *very* exposed! – and given a 'pre-med'. This may contain a mild sedative to make you relax but is mainly a chemical that dries up the saliva in your mouth, so you won't choke on it while under the anaesthetic. You will then be taken into the operating suite and, if having a general anaesthetic, sent to sleep. If you are having a local anaesthetic, the surgeon will freeze the relevant areas. Local anaesthesia is not used very often for a female sterilization, and then only if you are having a laparoscopic sterilization. This is probably the most popular method of sterilizing women in the Western world now and is the least traumatic or damaging way of entering the pelvic cavity.

An instrument called a trocar makes a puncture in the abdominal wall, in the umbilicus or naval. Through this is inserted the laparoscope. The laparoscope acts as a telescope and looks very much like one. It is a metal instrument that uses fibre optics to simultaneously shine a light into the body and pass back a clear picture to the operator. Some surgeons use a type of laparoscope that allows them to pass the instruments they need to do the operation down the laparoscope itself, so everything is done through the one hole. Others make a further cut in the abdominal wall, further down below the bikini line, insert a cannula or hollow tube into your pelvic cavity and pass the operating instruments down this.

Through the laparoscope the surgeon can get a good view of the pelvic cavity and all the organs squashed up against each other. To make the view easier two steps may be taken. First, the patient can be placed on a tilting bed with her head lower than her feet. This has the effect of allowing the digestive tract – the stomach itself and the coils of bowel – to shift slightly upwards inside the body. They then do not crowd down on or around the uterus and fallopian tubes, and this allows the surgeon to see and move these organs around more freely. To give further aid, a gas, usually carbon dioxide, is pumped inside before inserting the laparoscope. By 'blowing up' the cavity, this lifts the stomach wall itself away from all the organs and gives room to separate every organ from those next to it.

The laparoscope is an expensive and complicated instrument and experience is needed for it to be used competently by a surgeon. Some doctors prefer to approach the fallopian tubes by more direct means and in some cases this is necessary. In the mini-laparotomy, a small cut is made low in the abdomen. Instead of going inside to do the sterilization, the surgeon brings the fallopian tubes outside. An instrument is inserted into the uterus via the vagina and an assistant gently twists this around. The uterus and the fallopian tubes are moved so that, in turn, they come below the cut made in the abdominal wall. Forceps are used gently to separate the tubes from the surrounding tissue and a small segment of each is pulled out of the pelvic cavity. They can then be blocked by whatever method is chosen before being returned inside and the cut closed with stitches. A surgeon can, of course, perform a sterilization by opening up your abdomen fully and entering to do the necessary procedures inside. This may be done when there is an incision being made already; for instance, for a caesarean delivery.

In some cases, a sterilization is performed through the vaginal wall. This is done when it is particularly important for there to be no abdominal scar or when there is a difficulty in going through the abdominal wall – such as when the patient is very overweight or already heavily scarred. An incision or puncture is made high in the

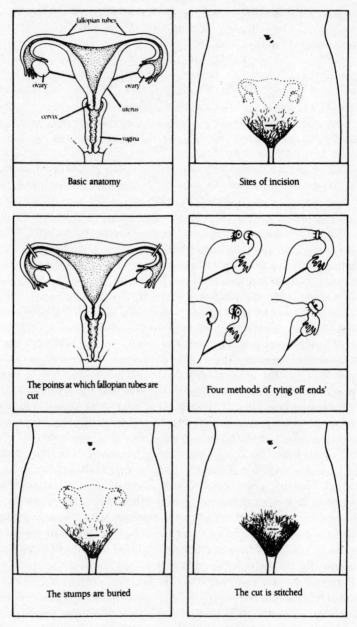

Figure 3 Female sterilization

vagina and a laparoscope passed through. However, vaginal incisions carry a higher risk of infection and are generally only used at present for good medical reasons.

The surgeon then has several choices as to how the tubes are to be prevented from carrying eggs down to the womb in future. They can be cut and the ends tied off or ligated. They can be cut, a section removed and the ends tied off. The cut ends can be doubled over on themselves or buried in surrounding tissue. A tiny plastic bag can even be sewn over the end of the tubes. They can be cauterized or burnt using an electrical instrument called a diatherm. Or they can be blocked using rings or clips that compress a section of the tube. Each method has its own particular pros and cons.

The ligatures or ties are not designed to remain intact – if they did, tissue would actually be encouraged to recanalize or form a tube again. They are there to stop bleeding and to persuade the cut ends of the tubes to close over. Plain catgut is used that dissolves within 72 hours. The ends of the tubes sometimes open again anyway, hence the risk of pregnancy later. Probably the safest methods are to remove the tubes entirely – a salpingectomy – or to use cauterization or diathermy. In cauterization or diathermy, a heat source is applied to the tube. This has the effect of burning out a section and simultaneously closing off the ends. The tube can also be cut and the ends diathermized. The entire blood supply in the fallopian tube can be coagulated or clotted by the procedure. This makes it almost impossible for the tube to heal itself and to allow you to fall pregnant afterwards. However, there are drawbacks in these two procedures. If you *did* change your mind and ask for a reversal operation, diathermy and salpingectomy leave very little or nothing for surgeons to work with. A surgeon, therefore, may only want to use these techniques if you are in your late thirties or forties and there is very little chance of your undergoing a change of heart.

The latest, and increasingly the most popular, method of blocking or occluding the fallopian tubes is using small devices in the shape of clips or rings. Fallope rings are tiny rings made of silastic (a type of plastic) which are put on the tubes with an applicator. A section of the fallopian tube is hooked and drawn up and the ring slides down over the hook, trapping the pulled up section. The trapped section is not only blocked off so sperm and eggs cannot pass through it, it also becomes hardened and lifeless.

Hulka and Filshie clips are made of plastic and metal. Hulka clips look like tiny crocodile jaws. Once applied, they crush the tube closed between the two plastic-toothed jaws, holding the tube squashed flat. Hulka clips can damage the tube so that even if they work loose or are removed the remaining scar tissue still may leave the tube blocked. Filshie clips are designed to be less harmful. Their jaws are smooth – metal-lined with a soft silastic insert. Although they hold the tube closed, if removed they leave less destruction than the Hulka clip. However, any damage caused by these methods is quite restricted, so a skilled surgeon might be able to restore fertility. If you have any inkling of a possible change of mind, these are the methods to request.

After blocking the tubes, the surgeon would close the opening to your pelvic cavity. The hole made by a trocar is only one to one and a half centimetres in diameter. One tiny stitch or clip may be used and the stitch may be buried in your skin so you can't even see it. Most surgeons use stitches that dissolve on their own although others prefer to use material that will need to be removed. You may have to go back to the hospital a week or so later for this or see your own GP.

If your operation was done under local anaesthetic, you are likely to be allowed to go home soon after. A general anaesthetic, however light, tends to make many people feel weak, dizzy or even sick. So after this you may need to lie down for a few hours or stay overnight to let you sleep it off. You may also be asked to stay overnight just to make sure that there are no difficulties or complications after the operation. Anaesthetists are getting better and better at using very light doses and since the pre-med used in these operations doesn't always contain a sedative, many patients feel little or no after effects from this operation. When you do go home, however, let someone else drive or otherwise look after you. Even small operations can leave you feeling a bit shaky.

Each method of opening the abdomen and of blocking off the tubes has its advantages and disadvantages. Opening up the body gives the surgeon the opportunity to see clearly all parts of the patient's pelvis and internal organs. With such a view, any unexpected problems such as fibroids or cysts can be picked up, and mistakes, such as confusing a ligament with a fallopian tube, will be avoided. The drawback is that you would have to recover from a fairly extensive procedure, needing several days in hospital, and be left with a scar. Open abdominal surgery is not exactly a method of choice nowadays. It is used when other methods are impossible, such as when the woman in question is *very* overweight or if her stomach is already heavily scarred from previous surgery. Women who are ileostomy or colostomy patients are also unable to be sterilized using the less intrusive methods.

Some doctors also take advantage of surgery to sterilize a patient when her abdomen has been opened for other reasons such as for a caesarean birth, or to perform surgery when she is in hospital for a period anyway, such as after childbirth. However, this does have one major drawback. The fallopian tubes are affected by pregnancy and are enlarged, friable and heavy with veins at this time. Performing any surgery or other procedure on them in this state is fraught with technical difficulties. The risk of the sterilization failing and a pregnancy occurring later is more likely at this point than at any other time. The blood supply to the tubes is so rich, that recanalization may well happen. Just as important is the fact that childbirth is possibly the worst time for an individual or couple to decide to opt for a sterilization. It may seem the best thing at the time, in the heat of the emotional upheaval and confusion of a new addition to the family, but feelings about this can change. Even if you accept that the child should be the last as well as the latest, you may not be happy to have that decision made irrevocable. And with the risks of cot death and the fact that children *do* still die in infancy, there is a chance you might regret a hasty decision. Being operated on at the time of an abortion may be even worse. In the now uncommon case of a surgeon trying to blackmail you into having a sterilization by making it a condition of giving you an abortion, resist strenuously. Nobody has the right to do this and another doctor is likely to help you without making such an unreasonable demand.

Although some methods are intrinsically better and less likely to fail than others, the skill of the individual surgeon is also important. A practised and experienced surgeon using a favourite but less effective method is less likely to have a patient become pregnant than an inexperienced surgeon using a 'fail-safe' method, or even an old hand trying out a different method for the first time.

What happens during a vasectomy?

A vasectomy is altogether a simpler operation. This is because men carry most of their reproductive organs outside the body. The tube that carries sperm from the testicles to the penis can be found just under the surface of the scrotum, making it very easy to isolate and divide. Vasectomy is almost always done under a local anaesthetic. In some clinics, a general anaesthetic is still offered, but unless there is a particular reason for this to be necessary, such as a terror of needles or operations or a difficulty in locating the vas, it is not advisable. Having a general anaesthetic is always a risk, however small, and there seems little point in exposing yourself to this risk if it is not needed. The local anaesthetic used will mask totally all sensation and make it a painless experience. If you like, you can even watch the operation. If you don't have the necessary suppleness to crane your neck enough to see, most doctors don't mind having a nurse hold a mirror so you can observe what is going on!

You will be asked to shave around your genitals and to arrive at the surgery, clinic or hospital fresh from a bath and with clean underwear. Boxer shorts, or no shorts at all, may be fashionable or preferred by you, but you should have a pair of snug fitting briefs or an athletic support or jock strap for after the operation.

You will be asked to lie down on a surgical table. This is usually tilted slightly so that your head will be lower than your feet in case of your feeling faint during the operation as is quite common. You will be covered with surgical sheets (they are usually deep green) with only your scrotum left exposed. Your penis will be tucked up, out of sight and harms way, under the sheet. You may feel horribly vulnerable and not a little silly. Surgeons try very hard not to approach with the syringe containing the local anaesthetic saying the usual, comforting statement, 'Don't worry, it's just a little prick.' It is worth pointing out here that most men are terrified at the idea that their surgeon might be a woman. This is partly because of a common masculine fear of the castrating female – the woman who will cut away your manhood – but also from the anxiety that she may laugh at your equipment, or even that you may disgrace yourself by having an erection at the wrong moment. She won't, and you won't. And even if you do shrink away to nothing from fear or stiffen slightly, be assured that she will not be alarmed, embarrassed or annoyed and *has* seen it all before!

Having cleansed the skin of the scrotum with an antiseptic liquid, the surgeon will begin the operation. The right side is usually done first. The surgeon will palpate or probe with the flats of his or her fingers to find the vas deferens. There are other structures in this part of the body that are also thin and cord-like, so this is not as easy as it sounds. When the surgeon is satisfied that the right part is between his or her fingers, the local anaesthetic will be injected

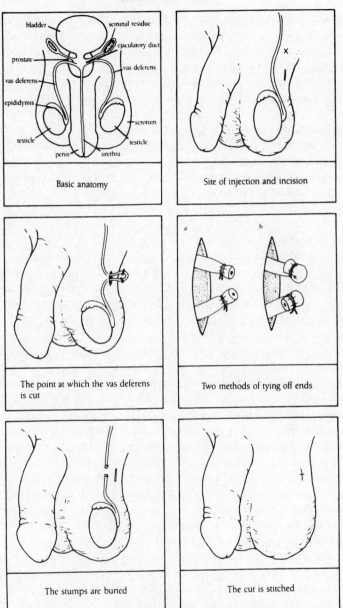

Figure 4   Vasectomy

under the skin and alongside the vas, to freeze the area that will be exposed and cut. After the anaesthetic has taken effect, after a minute or so, a lengthwise incision is made and the vas found and pulled out. The surgeon will put two clamps on the exposed loop and cut out the section in between. The ends are then tied with absorbent catgut and the vas is often turned over on itself and tied again.

Sometimes a section is not cut out but the two ends are tied together with the cut ends facing opposite directions. Or, after cutting, the cut ends are cauterized or diathermized to seal them. The stumps are then buried back in the tissue of the scrotum and the incision sewn up. Absorbent catgut is used for this by some doctors, while others prefer to use black silk, which will have to be removed later when the wounds have healed. The whole procedure is repeated on the opposite side. To finish, the area around each cut is cleansed, dried and covered with a plaster or gauze.

Some surgeons prefer to make *one* incision lengthwise down the centre of the scrotum, feeling for and pulling each vas in turn through this. The obvious advantage is there is only then one cut to heal. However, some doctors feel that having to pull the vas over to the centre can cause unnecessary damage to surrounding tissue. It also increases the chances of mistaking another cord for the vas and cutting or blocking the wrong object. Some surgeons make crosswise rather than lengthwise incisions.

Quite a few men have attacks of faintness during the operation, usually because of stress and fear. You might find you feel sick and have difficulty in breathing. If you begin to feel strange, tell the doctor immediately so he or she can remove the scalpel in case you start flailing about. The doctor or assistant will probably put a cold compress on your forehead and ask you to breathe deeply for a few minutes until you feel better. If you *do* faint, and again this is not uncommon, you will wake up again in a few seconds and be helped to breathe deeply until the dizziness and nausea go away.

After the operation, you may feel weak and faint and most clinics will provide a cup of tea or coffee (nothing stronger!) which will perk you up. Attacks of faintness or difficulty in breathing can come later, which is why being driven home, rather than driving yourself, is a good idea. Quite apart from the actual distress and danger of a crash, you may find your insurance will not cover you in the day following an operation.

Case histories

Martin's and Helen's story

Martin had a vasectomy after the birth of their third child. 'Several friends had had the op and I'd heard about it. Two of them said it didn't hurt at all, but one said he couldn't walk for a week, so I was a bit nervous when the day came.' The most alarming aspect from his point of view was that the surgeon turned out to be a woman. 'I hadn't expected that! The doctors I'd seen in the clinic before were men and it never occurred to me to ask. On the day itself, the doctor on duty was female and if Helen hadn't been with me, I might have done a runner.'

Martin found the nurses extremely helpful and matter-of-fact. Any embarrassment and fright he did have melted away under their approach. 'I suppose it's a bit like going to the dentist and it's never as bad as you think it's going to be. Mind you, you do feel a bit of a fool. They put these sheets over you, and there's your equipment, sort of lying out in the open and looking very small and insignificant. But the whole thing is over so quickly. I tried to watch at first and then felt a bit faint, so I put my head back and closed my eyes. When I opened them again to look, the doctor said it was all over.'

Martin took his doctor's advice after the operation. Helen drove them home and he rested for the whole weekend. 'The only problem was our little one kept wanting to sit on my lap and kept forgetting why I found this painful! And the cat was even more of a nuisance. Helen caught her in mid-leap a couple of times. I had some good bruises to show the next week, I can tell you.'

Nick's and Janet's story

Janet had her operation a year after the birth of her second child. 'We did ask for it while I was pregnant, but my doctor said I should wait until Ben was at least a year old. She explained why, and I could see the sense even though we were sure our minds were made up.' Janet found having to stay in hospital was a chore to arrange. 'My sister came and stayed, and Nick was very good. When it actually came round, having to stay in the hospital and be looked after for three days was bliss.' Janet found hospital routine was quite a relief after the busy life of a wife, mother and part-time teacher. 'Meeting other women in the same situation was fun, and we all compared reactions after the operations.'

She had expected to find the operation incisions painful and was surprised how little they hurt after she woke up. 'But I did feel so blown-up, and had a bad attack of the wind the next day. I hadn't expected that. I also did too much; I felt so relieved and happy that I rushed around like a mad thing. I then suddenly felt faint and dizzy, and the staff found me sitting on the floor with my head between my knees. I got told off for not being careful. It's surprising how much it can take out of you even though it does leave such a little mark.'

5

After the operation

I drove myself home after my vasectomy and a few miles outside our village I realized the car was getting rather hot. It was a Reliant Scimitar with a fibreglass body which I had spent hours restoring. I stopped, got out and like an idiot opened the bonnet. The engine was on fire and the whole lot went up in flames, melted and ran down the gutter. There I was, standing having had the chop, with my beloved car in ruins. It really was adding insult to injury – two symbols of my masculinity gone in one day. Still I can laugh about it now and truthfully say I don't regret it. The vasectomy, that is!

Philip C

It has been said that having a vasectomy takes about the same time as having your hair cut and need be no more traumatic! Male and female sterilizations *are* quick and easy operations, and there is no reason for you to be worried or afraid of the operation itself or the after effects. Serious complications are extremely rare. It is, however, important that you know what you are likely to find and experience, as well as what *could* happen. If there is a genuine problem you will be aware of it and seek help at once. So, how will you feel after your sterilization, and what are the danger signs?

After female sterilization

You are likely to feel bruised and in a bit of pain after the operation. However gentle your surgeon has been, cutting through tissue and manipulating instruments inside you is still bound to pressure and damage tissue. If you have had a general anaesthetic, you may feel drowsy for some hours after your awakening and feel sick. While you were under the general anaesthetic, the anaesthetist would have passed an instrument called an endotrachial tube down your throat. This is designed to hold your air passage open and free of obstruction so that you can breathe even when deeply unconscious. To pass the tube down, the anaesthetist will have had to tip your head right back and this can put some strain on your neck muscles. You may well find that you have shoulder-tip pain – an ache in the hollows of your shoulder above the collar bones – for a day or so after the operation. Your throat may also feel raw and sore, especially when swallowing.

As well as feeling battered around the abdominal area, you may be troubled by a bloated sensation and could have wind. The gas pumped into you to separate the organs and make the operation easier can contribute to both these feelings. Most of this gas would have been allowed to escape from the puncture or incision openings before they were closed up, but some may remain. This will be absorbed by your tissues fairly quickly and cannot harm you. Any discomfort will go eventually. Your digestive systems may also have been upset by the operation and the fact that you had to fast before it. As well as the actual incision being tender and bruised, sometimes you can also develop a haemotoma – a swelling caused by blood leaking into surrounding tissue at the puncture sites.

Complications after a sterilization operation are rare, but when they do occur can be quite serious. If blood vessels are not closed off properly, undetected bleeding in the pelvic cavity can be very damaging. Burns or cuts on the bowel can lead to a leakage of material into the cavity, and infection even leading to gangrene. *Very* occasionally, surgeons can damage the bowel or puncture large blood vessels, either with the needle used to pump in gas or with the device used to make the hole for the laparoscope. Just as rarely, they may touch the metal of the laparoscope while diathermizing the tubes, heating it and burning loops of the bowel. It is even possible to puncture the aorta or main artery in the body. This would be an unmistakeable accident as blood would spray everywhere and the damage would be repaired at once. Puncturing or damaging the bowel can sometimes be missed. In such an extremely rare situation, the undetected damage could lead to an infection and inflammation of the lining of the pelvic cavity called peritonitis. Peritonitis can take some days to develop. So, if you experience discomfort and pain within fifteen days of having a sterilization, make sure the doctor is aware of your distress.

Another cause of abdominal pain after such an operation is ectopic pregnancy. This is where a fertilized egg becomes lodged and starts developing somewhere other than in the uterus. The most dangerous and also the most likely place for this to happen is in the fallopian tubes. The tubes can only stretch so far and after a short time will rupture, causing extensive bleeding. As well as pain in the abdominal area, an ectopic pregnancy might give you referred pain around the collar bone. So again, if you have pain and discomfort that does not decrease or that gets worse, let your doctor know immediately and don't be fobbed off. Both of these conditions can be serious and can even lead to death if they are ignored. But please remember that such events are *very* rare.

If a sterilization fails, pregnancy is likely to occur in the first year after your operation. Although failures *are* unusual, they do happen. So, if you experience symptoms you recognize as being those of pregnancy, don't discount them just because you have had the operation. Between one and five women in every thousand will find that her sterilization has failed. Failures are more likely to happen if your operation was carried out by a surgeon who does few sterilizations, or if the doctor was trying out a technique new to them. If the operation followed immediately on an abortion or childbirth, you are also more at risk of its failing.

Even the most experienced surgeon can make mistakes. In the mass of tissue and ligaments that confronts a surgeon when he or she looks into the pelvic cavity, it is relatively easy to pick on the wrong object. When you see internal organs displayed in a diagram, they are clear, separate and often labelled. In their natural state, they can be squashed out of shape, pushed out of the usual place and be very similar in size, texture and colour to an entirely different bit. Surgeons can cut, block or put clips or rings on ligaments instead of tubes, or even burn or cut the ureters (the tubes that carry your urine or waste water) or sections of the bowel. A clip or ring may not have been put on securely and only close off part of a tube, or be thrown off by the organs' natural movements. Internal organs do move around quite a lot. Although they are tethered in place by ligaments they are not fixed immovably. Such mistakes are inexcusable, but they are at least understandable.

Pregnancies can also occur after a sterilization because they had actually begun *before* the operation. It is now fairly common practice for surgeons to perform a D and C, or Dilatation and Curretage (the widening of the cervical canal and the scraping out of the womb lining), as the final act in a sterilization. This is done just in case a pregnancy had already begun but not yet shown, or if a fertilized egg is on its way down the end section of the tube and approaching the womb. The lining having been removed, an egg will find no opportunity to embed and begin to develop. However, if an egg had actually been at its earliest stage of development, and had been trapped in the top section and cut off from being able to proceed down to the uterus, it might become an ectopic pregnancy. For this reason, newly sterilized women may be advised to pay particular attention to any symptoms that could suggest such an event. This is why it is important to use a method of birth control right up to the time you have the operation.

A side effect of sterilization that could be a minor annoyance or a major irritation is increased and painful periods. A sterilization does not stop you having periods – your womb is still intact and the hormones that drive your menstrual cycle are still produced and passed around your body as before. There has been much discussion about this link in the last few years. Women's complaints of heavier periods often have been discounted by many doctors. Their explanation was that, rather than the operation bringing about any change in menstrual patterns, it was perception and memory that was at fault.

Another explanation was that patterns were altered by other factors. Many women who are being sterilized are coming off the Pill for the first time in years. The periods you have while you are on the combined Pill are far lighter than periods you would have when not using hormonal contraception. It could be that a woman who feels her periods become heavier after a sterilization has just forgotten how heavy her periods had been before she used the Pill. Women having sterilizations are also likely to be older than the average woman using any other method of contraception, and since periods can alter and grow heavier towards the menopause, this may also lead to their having heavier bleeds.

However, a recent study showed that among women having an hysterectomy for abnormal bleeding, three times as many had been sterilized as had not. This and other recent studies appear to indicate that a sterilizing operation in itself *can* lead to heavier periods. The interference in the blood flow to the ovaries might have some feedback effect on the hormonal balance and on the growth and shedding of the lining of the womb. It would also seem that the greater the damage to tissue at the time of the operation, the more likely and the more extreme the symptoms. Thus, a woman having a diathermy is more likely to have heavier periods later than one sterilized by clips or rings. Also, individual surgeons seem to produce different results. Some are more likely to have patients who complain of this problem than others. It would appear that as well as using techniques that produce less tissue damage, some doctors have a defter touch than others.

The first and most important question that pops into your mind after the operation, however, is probably, 'Do I still feel as sexy and am I as desirable as I was?' The firm answer is that the sterilization operation itself has no dampening affect on your sexual urges or your attractiveness or femininity. Indeed, doctors will almost certainly tell you that it has no effect whatsoever. However, studies have shown that newly sterilized couples tend to make love *more often* after their operation than they did before.

The reason for this is open to debate. It may be that freedom from the anxiety of an unwanted pregnancy allows couples to have sex when previously they may have felt inhibited. Another explanation is that newly sterilized individuals feel under pressure to prove that the operation has *not* taken away their masculinity or femininity. To show themselves and their partners that this has not happened, they may throw themselves into lovemaking with renewed enthusiasm. Whatever the reason, you can at least be assured that blocking your tubes has no effect on the production and circulation through your body of the hormones that help make you sexually interested. Indeed, sexual feelings are just as much a matter of attitude and emotion as hormones anyway! A female sterilization won't make you put on weight (so if this happens to you, you'll have to find another excuse – you can't blame your operation!) or make you age ahead of your time. Since the ovaries are left untouched and go on producing their hormones, you do not have a premature menopause.

Female sterilization is effective from the moment the surgeon blocks those tubes, so as soon as you feel like making love, you are safe to do so. You may want to leave it a week or so until your abdomen feels less tender, or to use the woman-on-top position, to relieve pressure on delicate tissue. You will find that the operation scars do fade quite quickly. The bikini cut of a mini-laparotomy may be hardly noticeable after some months when your pubic hair has grown back. The puncture sites for a laparoscope may be so small that you would have to search for them the following year.

After vasectomy

When the anaesthetic wears off, you will probably feel bruised and sore. Wearing good support, even when lying down or sleeping, will help, and you should do this for at least the first 48 hours (and advisedly for a week) after, day *and* night. This lifts your scrotum and relieves pressure on the bruised tissue. The area must also be kept dry, so bathing or washing the scrotum should be avoided for the first three days or so. After this, soak the dressings off in a bath, but be careful to dry the site thoroughly (a hair dryer is the best way to do this well and painlessly). Put on another plaster and have at least one bath daily until both cuts are completely healed and the stitches have dissolved or come out.

The wounds may heal cleanly or they may ooze a clear liquid, that dries to a crusty yellow, for the next week. This is quite common – around one in ten men experience it – especially around the time that dissolving stitches are working themselves free. Keep the area clean and put a handful of salt into your bathwater. If wounds do become reddened or ooze thick yellow matter – pus – see your doctor at once. You would probably be prescribed antibiotics to clear up any infection. This is unusual, however. You are likely to find a hard, pea-sized swelling through the scrotal wall, over the cut ends of the vas. This will remain, is normal, usually painless and nothing to worry about. Most of the time these are not troublesome, and you will only notice it if you probe.

If you are sensible enough to examine your own testicles regularly for bumps and lumps to catch any signs of cancer, cysts or other problems before they become dangerous, you will find these lumps and be able to distinguish them from any other potentially dangerous swellings. Sometimes, however, these lumps, called a sperm granuloma, are a bother. They are caused by sperm leaking from the cut end of the vas into the surrounding tissue and setting up a reaction. Very occasionally, nerves become trapped in them and they become tender or ache. If they are persistently troublesome, you can have them removed by surgery.

Some people feel well enough to drive or even to go back to work soon after the operation, but the best advice is to take it easy, be driven home by somebody else and to put your feet up for the next 24 to 48 hours. The more you are on your feet and the more effort you exert, the more risk there is of your suffering a haemotoma. This is a tender swelling caused by blood seeping into tissue – a glorified bruise, in fact. Large haemotomas may be painful and obstructive enough to need a hospital admission for them to be drained.

Most vasectomies will give rise to some bruising and certainly to tenderness. You might expect bruising directly around the operation site, but also be prepared for it to extend some way beyond this region. The seeping blood that causes a bruise can drain some way through tissue, discolouring your flesh over quite an area. If streaks and pools of bruising reach up to your navel or down your thighs, do not be surprised or alarmed. However, try not to have your vasectomy just before going away on a summer holiday, or you could attract some alarmed glances on the beach, especially if it's a nudist one!

As well as discolouring, the scrotum itself may swell slightly and appear puffy. The swellings may be painless, could come up above one or both testicles, and can be as large as the testicle itself. This is caused by a temporary blockage in the lubricating fluid surrounding the testicle and will drain away in time. However, if the swelling is noticeable, don't just be delighted at this apparent increase in your credentials, do see your doctor as you may well have to have it drained. For all these reasons, it is often best to arrange for your vasectomy just before a two- or three-day break from work, so you can give yourself the chance to recuperate in peace. The wounds will heal with very little scarring, which may even be hidden among the folds of your scrotal sac. Unless she looked very carefully indeed a partner may not even be able to see where you have been cut.

Perhaps even more than women, men are intensely concerned about their sexual prowess after a vasectomy. You may be somewhat eager to make love as soon as possible after the operation, to see if there is any difference. You are most unlikely to be able to detect any. Your ability to become excited, to become erect, to experience orgasm will all be as before. After a vasectomy, your body continues to manufacture sperm as it did before. However, instead of progressing up the vas to an exit, the maturing cells are absorbed back into the body with no harmful effects. The orgasm itself will feel the same, and the amount and appearance of ejaculate you produce will seem unchanged. Only two per cent of potent ejaculate is sperm, the rest is semen or lubricating and nourishing fluid.

If anything, you are likely to notice an improvement, but this is probably all in the mind. An explanation for male sexual interest after a vasectomy is that sperm-producing and hormone-producing cells in the testes might undergo a change following the operation. It has been suggested that the sperm-producing cells may be damaged and decrease, but that the cells that produce secretions and hormones (the Leydig cells) might increase in volume. If so, this would suggest a slightly higher secretion of hormones that *could* increase a man's sex drive. The evidence is by no means certain, and it is not a good reason for asking for a sterilization.

Contrary to any scare stories you might have heard, vasectomy does not lead to impotence, premature ageing or to any other form of physical ill health. There have been some studies that appear to suggest that such ill effects could result from this operation. Don't let them put you off. These studies have all been carried out on animals such as monkeys which, although they may have some resemblance to human beings, *are* different. Some research appears to show an association between prostate cancer and cigarette smoking, early sexual intercourse, a family history of disease and vasectomy. However, in the largest on-going study done on human beings, no ill effects have been noted as a result of the operation. Indeed, vasectomized men appear to be healthier and to live longer than their unvasectomized counterparts. Nobody is making any magic claims for the power of vasectomy from this. It is probable that the explanation is that the sort of man who has a vasectomy is also the sort of man to have a healthy lifestyle. Cutting the channel that enables sperm to travel to the outside world has only *one* result, that of blocking the cells that could combine with cells from a woman to start a pregnancy.

Vasectomized men do not run a risk of becoming impotent – not from the effects of the operation, that is. If you do have sexual problems, they might arise from your fears and beliefs about the operation, but it will not be the vasectomy that has done this to you. Vasectomy has no effect on the production of the chemicals that fuel a man's sexual urges. These are still manufactured in the testicles and absorbed – as they would be *before* a vasectomy – into the bloodstream and thence sent around the body. The vas deferens is never involved in this exchange. Similarly, the mechanism by which sexual interest is turned into action – an erection – is also unaffected. Cutting this channel does not cut off the blood supply to the penis, which is how you have an erection. Men afraid of being damaged by someone 'mucking around with the family jewels' should be reassured by a basic understanding of how their body works.

The only physical effect of a vasectomy relates to your chances of a reversal. The absorbtion back into the body of sperm cells does appear to set up a reaction in the immune system in around half the men who have the operation. This does not *damage* the immune system in any way, let us hasten to add. What it does is alert your body to your own sperm and begin to treat them as a foreign, harmful substance. After a time, the immune system works to detect and neutralize any sperm found in the body. This includes in the testicles. You will still be as virile and as sexy as before, but even if a successful reversal operation were performed, you may find that your sperm are now unable to impregnate (start a pregnancy).

You may not feel like making love for a week or so until any swelling or tenderness has gone. Then again, you may. You can resume making love when you feel comfortable. It is suggested, however, that you wait a week or so before you do this. One warning to be written in letters of fire above your bed; A VASECTOMY IS *NOT* IMMEDIATELY EFFECTIVE. It will take up to about 36 ejaculations before all the sperm left in the vas above the blocked area have been flushed out of your body. So in most cases, a vasectomy is not going to be an effective method of contraception for three to four months after you have had the operation. Of course, the sooner and the more you make love, the quicker you will be safe. Until you have had *two* clear sperm counts (that is, free of *all* sperm), one after the other, checked by your doctor, go on using another method of birth control.

Some doctors now wash out the vas by flushing a flow of sterile water through the part that continues from the scrotum out through the penis. Even so, some viable sperm can remain in this section after the operation. The ejaculate will appear identical before and after a successful vasectomy – you cannot tell by looking at it with the naked eye whether you are clear or not. It is best not to trust to vague estimates, but to have a semen analysis and wait for two consecutive clear sperm counts before trusting to the success of the operation.

It is worth noting in this context that having had a vasectomy will not in any way protect you from catching a sexually transmitted disease or from passing one on. If viruses such as those that cause AIDS or Herpes, and the organisms that cause NSU, Gonorrhoea or other diseases are present, they would not only be in the sperm, but in *all* body secretions. They will be present in semen even if sperm is no longer travelling from the testicles along the vas.

Vasectomies fail less often than female sterilizations – around one in a thousand men will cause a pregnancy afterwards. So it is rare, but by no means unheard of. If the partner of a vasectomized man becomes pregnant, surgical failure rather than infidelity could be the reason. In some cases, the vas was missed and a spermatic cord divided instead. In others, but very rarely, a third vas exists and is missed. More frequently, the body repairs itself and the vas rejoins. This is called recanalization. Since sperm are driven by pressure rather than, as in the female, the wavelike action of the cilia lining the tube, the actual state of the pathway is immaterial. As long as a passage exists sperm can get through. In some cases, sperm will even travel through the tissue across a gap between the cut and separate ends of the vas. Recanalization, if it is to occur, usually happens fairly quickly after the operation. As long as you have had two consecutive zero sperm counts – and *only* after you have had this confirmation – you would usually be safe. However, authenticated cases of recanalization have been reported as late as ten years after a vasectomy. So again, if the symptoms of pregnancy *do* occur, don't discount them but have a pregnancy test.

Both men and women might find the immediate after effects of a sterilizing operation cause some discomfort. Compared to the physical and emotional problems that could arise if you suffered an unwelcome pregnancy or struggled on with an alternative method of birth control that did not suit you, the annoyance may seem trivial and well worth it.

Case histories

Nick's and Terri's story

Nick was surprised at how little he noticed his vasectomy. He had very little bruising and not much discomfort. However, he did notice that a small, nagging ache developed inside his scrotum. It seemed to focus on a small lump that he could feel just under the incision site on one side. 'It seemed to get worse whenever we made love, although that could just have been because I was more aware of it at that time.' One night, Nick lost his erection as he and Terri were about to make love, and from then on he found himself avoiding lovemaking. This went on for some months.

Nick had his routine sperm counts, which remained positive. His doctor remarked on the fact that they should have become negative by now. 'He pointed out that either the vasectomy had failed or that we weren't making love very often. Well, I hadn't really liked to say anything, but I told him what had happened.' Nick had felt that the trouble was his fault, or that it was a side effect of vasectomy that could not be altered. In fact, his doctor explained that he obviously had a sperm granuloma which could be removed. Nick went back to the hospital for another, quick operation. This time the results were perfect. The nagging pain went and the couple resumed their former happy and enjoyable sex life.

Joyce's story

Joyce was delighted with her sterilization, but less happy when a year later she started to have heavy and painful periods. Some months the bleeding would come on so rapidly that she would find herself with soaked underpants. Even using a tampon and a sanitary towel would not be enough protection on the second and third days and she would have to change them every half hour or so. Her own doctor was dismissive and seemed to believe she was exaggerating until, in desperation, Joyce turned up at his surgery in full flood. He then referred her to the hospital, where she saw a different gynaecologist to the one who had done her sterilization. The new surgeon confirmed Joyce's impression – that periods *can* become heavier after a sterilization, especially if radical surgery had been used. Joyce had been sterilized by diathermy.

Once she was satisfied that it wasn't all in her mind, Joyce decided to put up with the symptoms for a few more months, but then asked for an hysterectomy. She made a good recovery from this. 'If I could make the choice again,' she says, 'I might have preferred to have had a sterilization with clips or to have had the tubes tied. I mean, I may have ended up needing to have an hysterectomy anyway, but it does seem that it was helped along by my operation, or so the doctor said.'

6

Reversals and failures

I shouldn't have had it, I knew I shouldn't have had it at the time. But he said he would leave me if I didn't get my tubes tied and like a fool I thought it would make all the difference. Well I suppose it did . . . he spent the two days I was in hospital fixing up to leave me and go off with her. I should be glad really because Brian is a very different kettle of fish and he's wonderful with the kids. Which is why I'd really like to give him one that will be ours.

Sheila D

One of the cardinal rules when seeking a sterilization is to consider the decision irrevocable. Once cut, fallopian tubes and the vas deferens are extremely difficult to reunite, and you should not go into the operation reassuring yourself that if it turns out you regret your decision, it can be reversed. However, one to three in every hundred of us who have been sterilized *will* return for an attempt at reinstating our fertility. Is a reversal possible?

Whether a reversal operation will eventually result in a pregnancy often depends on a combination of factors. These include:

- Your age, if you are a woman.
- The interval between being sterilized and seeking a reversal, if you are a man.
- The method used to sterilize you.
- The skill of the surgeon operating on you now.

Who asks for a reversal? The answer may serve as a warning if you are reading this while trying to make up your mind whether or not to be sterilized. People who request a reversal operation tend:

- to be under 50;
- to have been sterilized before they were 30;
- to have an unstable marriage or one that has broken up;
- to have had their sterilization soon after a pregnancy;
- to have had more problems with contraception before opting for sterilization than those who remain happy with the operation;
- to have a low income.

The last factor may be linked to the fact that people on low incomes may have had very little real choice or power in the sterilization decision. They may have allowed well-meaning doctors or social workers to persuade them to 'do the sensible thing' by forcibly limiting the size of their family and the number of their dependents. Two thirds of those requesting a reversal have a new marital partner and want to establish the bond of a child between them, however large their separate families already are. In one study, half the men who asked for reversals of a vasectomy were divorced or separated and 80 per cent of them had chosen as new partners women who did not already have a child.

You may be tempted to request a reversal of sterilization for other reasons. Some men and women feel inadequate and abnormal after a sterilization. Even though you might not want another child, you might find you need the *potential* to become a parent to feel normal. You might even find that lovemaking loses its savour and becomes meaningless if there is no possibility that a pregnancy could result. If you feel that way, then certainly speak to your doctor about the possibility of a reversal. But for those reading this before the event, if you have the slightest doubt that these emotions might trouble you, *don't* be sterilized!

Female sterilization reversal

Some surgeons claim extraordinarily good results for the reversal operation. In fact, the expertise of the reversing surgeon is less important than the skill or choice of method of the original doctor. Success depends on how and where on the fallopian tubes he or she operated and on the extent of the ensuing damage. In some cases, it isn't even worth attempting a reversal. Often those impressive figures are more a result of being very selective over which patients are accepted for reversal operations than actual medical genius with a scalpel. After all, if you reject all but the most hopeful cases, you can easily claim to have a high percentage of success. It has been claimed that among those considered suitable for a reversal operation, up to 80 per cent may have a successful pregnancy. However, other studies suggest that only ten to fifteen per cent of attempted reversals would be successful. Furthermore, ten per cent of subsequent pregnancies are ectopic, so although sperm can travel up the fallopian tube, the fertilized egg cannot travel down to the womb and becomes trapped partway.

If you request a reversal operation, the surgeon will need details of your original operation. Indeed, often the best option is for you to return to see the surgeon who sterilized you in the first place. If the method used was blocking by a clip or ring, or by the Pomeroy procedure, the doctor may decide to go ahead and attempt restoration without further ado. If a more destructive method was used, you may be admitted to hospital for an exploratory operation first. The surgeon would perform a laparoscopy, to examine your tubes and assess the damage to them. A reversal operation is a more serious undertaking than a sterilization. You would have to be unconscious for longer and the incision made for the surgeon to be able to do his or her work would almost certainly have to be larger. This means you will need to stay in hospital for longer afterwards, and have a bigger scar to heal.

Having entered your abdomen, the surgeon would remove the clips or rings from your fallopian tubes and/or delicately cut away any damaged or scarred portion of the tubes. Doctors *can* sterilize a woman with a mind to whether or not they will need to undo their work later on. Reversals are most difficult when the operation has affected the whole length of the fallopian tubes, as in diathermy, or has been toward one or the other end of the tubes – near the uterus itself (the cornual) or near the ovaries (the fimbrial part). In both of these positions, the tubes vary from a narrow section near the middle of the tubes outwards to a wider section. If the surgeon has to remove a damaged part and then try to align and sew together the remaining undamaged lengths, he or she will find that one side is noticeably larger than the other. Needless to say, this makes the job harder, if not impossible. If, however, the excised section or the section damaged by rings or clips was in the isthmal or central part, microsurgery could possibly reassemble a viable tube.

Tubes become blocked and lead to ectopic pregnancies for two reasons. First, damaged tissue tends to build up in an attempt at healing itself and this can result in a clumsy mass of scar tissue sticking the sides of the tubes to each other. Second, whether the central bore of the tube remains open or can be reinstated, the *lining* of that opening cannot be repaired. All along the inside of your fallopian tubes are tiny cells called cilia. They resemble little hairs or the tentacles on sea anemones. These cilia pulse gently together, setting up a current and flow of fluid from the ovaries, down the fallopian tubes to the womb. It is on this current that a maturing egg floats from the ovary on its journey to the womb. If the cilia are damaged, the egg's journey could be in fits and starts and it may lose momentum and become stranded *in* the tube. Damage towards the middle part of the tube is less likely to cause this sort of problem than damage at either end.

Another problem with reinstating tubes is that the length of the tube is an important factor in establishing a pregnancy. A fertilized egg needs to spend some seven days in its journey from the outer end of the tube and its meeting with sperm, to entering the womb and embedding in the lining. If a surgeon has to remove a considerable length of damaged tube, or a large section was originally cut out, this journey may be cut short. If so, the egg reaches the uterus too soon and cannot implant and is lost.

Needless to say, a reversal operation is only successful if both partners are still fertile anyway. As women get older fertility wanes, so it is possible for the operation itself to be a success but a pregnancy still not to arrive. Before having the operation, it is a good idea for your male partner to have a semen test to see whether he is fertile. This is a wise move even if he *has* already been a father.

Vasectomy reversal

In contrast, as many as 90 per cent of vasectomy reversals are successful in that the operation can restore a clear passage for the sperm to travel from the testicles to the outside world. However, the longer the interval between vasectomy and reversal, the greater the risk that your body will have set up an immune reaction to your own sperm and for it to have become sterile. For this reason, the expected pregnancy rate after vasectomy reversal is less – around 30 per cent.

As with the woman's operation, vasectomy reversal is a far more extensive procedure than vasectomy itself. It can be done under local anaesthesia, but since it can take some time a general anaesthetic is usually advised. After making an incision into the scrotum, the surgeon will trim away the cut and damaged ends of the vas. The surgeon will be looking for a flow of sperm from the section of vas still attached to the testicle. The tube may have become scarred, especially if it has been several years since the vasectomy. This may mean that a portion of vas may have to be cut away until the surgeon finds a clear passage. As with women, a shortening of the tube can produce problems, since sperm need a period of maturation. They grow from immaturity to full strength while travelling around the coiled channels in the testes – the epididymis. If the vas is seriously foreshortened, there is a possibility that the resultant sperm may be too immature to be viable. If you were vasectomized by having a section cut from the vas and the ends cauterized, you may present more of a challenge than if the vas was cut and the ends buried in tissue or tied side by side.

The operation is more likely than a vasectomy to leave you feeling battered and bruised, and to suffer a haematoma. Indeed, you may well find after you wake up that draining tubes have been left in the incision to prevent this happening. You will have to stay in hospital overnight after the procedure, and these will be removed the next day. You will have to take slightly more care of yourself after this operation than after the vasectomy. You don't want to risk sudden movements or strain, stretching your tissues and pulling the vas apart again. You would probably be told to add three or four days to everything in the original timetable – putting your feet up, not lifting, not going to work and not making love. At the end, the only physical difference you will be able to *see* will be slightly more noticeable scars.

Case histories

Graeme's and Dorothy's story

Graeme was delighted with his vasectomy, in spite of the fact that he did suffer some bruising and pain. He and Dorothy had always enjoyed their love life and lost no time in getting back to lovemaking soon after. Graeme attended for his sperm counts, but did find the experience off-putting. 'I had to produce a sperm sample for analysis and, as luck would have it, my mother had come to stay. There I was, clutching this bottle, wanting to get into the bathroom to do my bit in private, and she just wouldn't come out. Dorothy was saying "Mother, can Graeme use the bathroom because he has to keep a doctor's appointment?", and there she was saying "Well, he can go at the surgery, can't he?" It's a bit difficult telling your own Mum that you need the bathroom to have a wank! So I rushed off and had to go into a public toilet, and it was the most nerve-wracking and embarrassing experience of my life. I was convinced somebody would come banging on the door at any moment and it was gruesome.'

Graeme was so put off, that when the count came back negative, he 'forgot' to go for the second test. Seven months later, Dorothy missed a period, but thought no more about it until she was sick one morning. Sure enough, a test soon showed that she was pregnant. A sperm analysis revealed that Graeme was still, or had reverted to, producing live sperm. A second vasectomy revealed that one of the vas had recanalized. Graeme and Dorothy decided to continue with the pregnancy and to accept this third, unplanned child, but made sure that he kept his appointments until he was given two fully negative results after the second operation.

Jenny's story

Jenny had her sterilization soon after the birth of her son, her and her husband Keith's second child. Three years later, Keith and the boy were killed in a car accident. Jenny has since re-married, to an old friend who adores her daughter. However, Jenny was desperate to have a child between the two of them – preferably a son. Her doctor spent a long time discussing this need. Jenny was aware that she could not replace or call back either of them from the dead. But she really did feel that she would be happier if she could at least try to give Brian child of his own.

Fortunately, her operation had been by the Pomeroy procedure. A small section from the middle of her tubes had been removed. Her surgeon was able to rejoin the ends that were left. Jenny had several late and heavy periods which she thinks were early miscarriages. She then suffered an ectopic pregnancy, which resulted in one tube having to be removed. Thirteen months after her reversal operation, she missed a period and, this time, there were no further accidents. She and Brian have their longed-for son.

7

The future

If present trends continue it is not unreasonable to expect that sterilization will eventually be used by most people as their final method of birth control. Already, many couples and individuals are recognizing that different contraceptive methods suit different circumstances and times. Rather than plumping for one method of contraception and sticking to it throughout your life, swopping methods to suit your lifestyle, family size, health and taste will become the norm. Sterilization is the obvious method for couples and individuals who feel that their childbearing days are over.

Experimental methods seem to concentrate on two aspects that could make sterilization even more acceptable to more people in the future. One is to perfect easier and quicker ways of delivering a foolproof, irreversible operation, to make having a sterilization less traumatic. The other is to find methods of sterilizing both men and women that could be easily reversed, so that we could change our minds or even routinely use this as a non-permanent method of birth control.

One suggestion is to reduce the stress and trauma of surgery for women by inserting the necessary devices up through the vagina and uterus, instead of having to cut through the vaginal or abdominal wall. If these and other techniques could be perfected, women could be sterilized as easily and as quickly as men are now vasectomized. The problem here is being able to see well enough to manoeuvre the instruments, while still only using the one opening of the cervix to gain access to the uterus and the tubes.

Researchers are exploring alternative ways of stopping the meeting of egg and sperm, or the implantation of a fertilized egg. Work has been done with toxic materials. Chemicals are delivered into the fallopian tubes or to the womb, scarring and destroying their ability to allow a pregnancy to occur or continue. As with other failures, researchers keep coming up against the body's remarkable ability to heal itself. Other researchers are experimenting with a form of superglue. Adhesive is put in the fallopian tubes, forming a plug and gluing the sides together.

Similar methods are being researched for men, including the use of chemicals to scar the vas. Chemicals or liquids that form plugs could be injected through the scrotal wall, without any surgery needing to be done. A further line of enquiry is the insertion of a fine needle to administer electrocautery – burning with an electric current – again without the need to cut into the scrotum.

As well as trying to make irreversible sterilization quicker and better, researchers are attempting to come up with a safe method that *can* be reversed. Ceramic, silicone rubber, copper, polyurethane, plastic or silastic and stainless steel plugs have all been tried out, both in men and women. These block the fallopian tubes or vas but can be removed leaving little damage. A variant on these contains a valve or tap. When implanted, the channel is closed. Instead of removing the device if a return to fertility is desired, the channel is merely reopened.

So far, the failure rates for all these methods are unacceptably high. With new materials coming onto the market every year and new techniques being found, some could promise much for the future.

8

Some common questions

Will I still ejaculate after a vasectomy?

Yes, and to the naked eye the liquid produced after a vasectomy will appear no different to that produced before. Around 98 per cent of the ejaculate, or 'come', is actually a protective fluid produced by the seminal vesicles and the prostate gland. This seminal fluid contains proteins and sugars to nourish the sperm and help them on their way up through the woman's vagina and on to a rendezvous with an egg in her fallopian tubes.

Only 2 per cent of the teaspoon of liquid pushed out at male climax is actually sperm. So after a vasectomy the moment of orgasm is far from 'dry'. The ejaculate looks, feels and smells the same, and the man's pleasure is undiminished. Only by putting the fluid under a microscope can you see that it no longer contains the tiny, tadpole-like sperm – and 2 per cent of a teaspoon is a very small amount to notice is missing.

Will I still have periods?

If your operation was undertaken with the specific intention of sterilizing you, you will still have periods as normal. Periods only stop if the ovaries are removed and menopause is triggered off, or if the womb itself has been taken away.

Such an operation would only be done for good medical reasons. When the only aim is to prevent further pregnancies, the operation blocks or removes part of the fallopian tubes. This does nothing to prevent further periods.

After sterilization, the ovaries continue to respond to the hormones produced by the pituitary and hypothalamus glands and to produce their own hormones, driving the menstrual cycle. Periods and Pre-Menstrual Syndrome (PMS) can continue as before, which is why sterilization is *not* advised as a way of solving menstrual problems.

Do I have to be over 35 with three children to be offered a sterilization?

Not any more. It is true that some surgeons used to apply what was called the '120 Rule' – your age multiplied by your number of children had to be 120 or more before they would grant a sterilizing operation. Nowadays, doctors accept that younger people with smaller families can rationally decide that their families are complete, and mean it. Most doctors would only wish to be convinced that you *did* appreciate the irrevocable nature of the operation, had thought long and hard about it and were sure about your decision, before they agreed to help you.

Will I age faster if I have a vasectomy?

We have no real evidence to support this fear. There have been some studies on monkeys that seem to suggest that the operation itself can increase atherosclerosis – a thickening of the arteries which restricts blood flow. The mechanism appears to be that the immune reaction that often occurs in vasectomized subjects increases their risks of material clogging up the arteries. But human beings are not monkeys. None of the studies done on men have confirmed these results. Indeed, in the longest and largest study on humans who have had a vasectomy, involving 10,000 vasectomized men and 10,000 matched unvasectomized men, those who had had the operation were shown to be healthier.

Can I be sterilized if I am childless?

Childlessness itself is no bar. Most doctors would want anyone requesting a sterilization to show that they accept and understand the implications of the operation, and are unlikely to change their mind. Clearly, someone who has not had *any* children may later decide that they want at least one. Equally clearly, they may not. Most surgeons will now be willing to listen to each individual patient's request and argument. Some may be of the opinion that a person who has firmly decided not to have any children at all is *less* likely to change their mind than someone who has already demonstrated that being a parent is and has been important to them. But if you are under 30 and have no children most doctors would not advise sterilization.

What if my children die after my sterilization?

Clearly this is a question you need to consider carefully before you opt for an operation. If your feeling is that, in the event of a tragedy occurring, you would want to have another chance at raising a family, you really should think twice before being sterilized.

Sterilization reversals *are* a possibility, but it is unwise to depend on them if having children survive you is very important to you. You could, however, opt for vasectomy and bank a sperm sample as an insurance. You would be asked to produce two or three fresh samples of your sperm, by masturbation. These are divided into containers called straws, frozen and kept for you until needed. There are no facilities on the NHS to do this at present, but several charities and commercial organizations offer it for a reasonable fee. This may be around £165–175 to establish your deposit and store it for five years, and then around £15 a year after that.

If your feeling is that your living children are the only ones you would ever want and even if they died you would not wish to try again, then you might wish to continue with an operation.

Is the operation painful?

Not at the time. Local or general anaesthetics will ensure you don't feel a thing as the knife goes in. But, of course, any surgical event cuts through tissue and leaves a sore and bruised area for a time. A vasectomy can leave you feeling as if you have been kicked in the testicles for several days, depending on how much care you take of yourself after the operation. A female sterilization can be like an unpleasantly painful, crampy period. The only question to ask yourself is, 'Is this pain worth it?' For most people, the answer is Yes.

Is the operation dangerous?

Any operation has its risks, especially if a general anaesthetic is used. Are the risks worth it? In most cases, yes. The medical risks of pregnancy are greater, to say nothing of the emotional and financial strain an unplanned and unwanted pregnancy can put you under. Most important, you can minimize the risks that you might run from a sterilizing operation by making sure your surgeon is practised and experienced in the technique to be used, and that you follow carefully any advice for your own aftercare.

What sort of people have sterilizations?

All sorts. All classes, all educational levels, all ages, single people, married people, people with large families and people with no children. The only link is that having looked at the subject carefully and considered all the options, they decide that sterilization is for them.

Do many GPs offer vasectomies in their surgeries?

According to the Family Planning Association, between 12,000 and 15,000 vasectomies are performed each year by trained family doctors. Some do this for free under the NHS. However, they are not reimbursed for their costs by the NHS. Providing surgery can be an expensive business – surgical gloves and instruments, and their own and a nurse's time adds up. So most would want to see you as a private patient for this and charge. Fees could be around £100.

What happens to the egg or the sperm after a sterilization?

The human body is designed to cope with the odd bit of microscopic tissue floating around inside. Even before a sterilizing operation, not all viable sperm or eggs find their way to the outside world. If their passage is blocked off, they are reabsorbed by the body, naturally and harmlessly. This process is common and does not make you fat, old before your time or lacking in sexual urges.

After I have been sterilized, do I still need to have regular smear tests?

Yes, you most certainly do. In spite of the fact that you no longer need to visit your doctor to get contraception, you still should be using your own doctor or the family planning clinic to get cancer checks. A sterilization has stopped only one thing: the passage of an egg from your ovaries to the outside world. It prevents nothing else in your body changing or developing. If cells on your cervix are going to go through the pre-cancerous changes that herald carcinoma of the cervix, they will do so whether you have had a sterilization or not. An hysterectomy, which has the side effect of sterilizing you, may well entail removing your cervix and so excising one cancer black spot. But a normal sterilization leaves everything bar your tubes untouched. If you have regular cancer checks, these changes will be spotted and treatment can be given to cure totally the disease before it really takes hold, whether you have had a sterilization or not.

Men, too, should examine their testicles regularly for lumps that might mean testicular cancer. The chances of developing this are exactly the same after as before a vasectomy.

Will having a vasectomy make me any less of a man?

No. Having your vas cut is not the same as having a castration operation. *That's* the operation to remove the testes entirely. A vasectomy leaves everything intact, it just stops sperm from getting through to the outside world. Don't confuse virility with fertility. You can be virile – sexy and both willing and able to have sex – without being fertile – able to have or cause a pregnancy. Indeed, if appearing masculine is important to you, consider this: what could be more macho than being so confident about your masculinity that you can happily accept an operation to make you sterile? It could even become a new boast: 'Real Men do it without having to prove anything!'

If I did decide to have a sterilization privately would it be very expensive?

Whether you consider a private vasectomy cheap at the price or out of your bracket obviously depends on how much you can spare. A vasectomy at one of the birth control charities will set you back around £120, while a female sterilization costs around £320. If you live some distance from one of their clinics, you would also have to pay travelling expenses and perhaps an overnight stay. So, a slightly more expensive operation from a local private surgeon may be a better deal.

Some trained doctors do vasectomies in their own surgeries and can charge less. Certainly, you may be justified in arguing the cost if you are quoted a fee much in excess of those quoted here. However stretched your budget and limited your income, a sterilizing operation comes out at less than you would pay on a summer holiday and less than you might get in an average pay cheque. Considering the expense of having a child, it has to be a bargain.

Useful addresses

Advice and information on Vasectomy and Sterilization

Health Education Authority
Hamilton House
Mabledon Place
London WC1H 9TX
Telephone 071 387 9528
Produce many excellent free pamphlets and can recommend books on health care and health-related problems.

Family Planning Association
27–35 Mortimer Street
London W1N 7RJ
Telephone 071 636 7866
Publish a wide range of leaflets on all aspects of sexuality and birth control. Have a mail order service for books. They can give you the address of your local family planning clinic.

Women's Health Concern
PO Box 1629
London W8 6AU
Telephone 071 938 3932

and

Women's Health
52 Featherstone Street
London EC1Y 8RT
Telephone 071 251 6333
Voluntary organizations that can give you useful information and support on any aspect of women's health care and family planning.

Charities offering information and operations

BPAS (British Pregnancy Advisory Service)
Austy Manor
Wootton Wawen
Solihull
West Midlands B95 6DA
Telephone 0564 793225

and

Pregnancy Advisory Service
13 Charlotte Street
London W1P 1HD
Telephone 071 637 8962

and

Marie Stopes House
108 Whitfield Street
London W1P 6BE
Telephone 071 388 0662
Charitable organizations that offer vasectomy and female sterilization and reversal operations for a reasonable fee. They also have
helpful leaflets on the operations and can provide, or help you to
obtain, sperm banking.

Difficulties with your doctor

Patients Association
18 Victoria Park Square
London E2 9PF
Telephone 081 981 5676

and

Association of Community Health Councils
30 Drayton Park
London N5 1PB
Telephone 071 609 8405

Organizations offering advice and support to patients who have any
worries or complaints about or difficulties with any doctor or
member of the medical profession.

Counselling and support

British Association for Counselling
1 Regent Place
Rugby
Warwicks CV21 2PJ
Telephone 0788 578328/9

and

Relate
Herbert Gray College
Little Church Street
Rugby CV21 3AP
Telephone 0788 73241

and

Catholic Marriage Advisory Council
Clitherow House
1 Blythe Mews
Blythe Road
London W14 0NW
Telephone 071 371 1341
Organizations which can offer, or direct you to, counselling to help
you make up your mind about whether to have a sterilization or not.

Further reading

Peter Bromwich and Tony Parsons, *Contraception: The Facts*, Oxford University Press 1990.

Dr Elizabeth Clubb and Jane Knight, *Fertility: A Comprehensive Guide to Natural Family Planning*, David and Charles 1992.

Dr Anna M. Flynn and Melissa Brooks, *A Manual of Natural Family Planning*, Unwin Paperbacks 1990.

John Guillebaud, *The Pill*, Oxford University Press 1991.

Julia Mosse and Josephine Heaton, *The Fertility and Contraception Book*, Faber and Faber 1990.

Paul Brown and Carolyn Faulder, *Treat Yourself to Sex*, Penguin Books 1989.

Michael Castleman, *Making Love*, Penguin Books 1988.

Alex Comfort, *The New Joy of Sex*, Mitchell Beazley 1991.

Gill Cox and Sheila Dainow, *Making the Most of Loving*, Sheldon Press 1988.

Gill Cox and Sheila Dainow, *Making the Most of Yourself*, Sheldon Press 1985.

Tony Gough, *Couples Arguing*, Darton, Longman and Todd 1987.

Suzie Hayman, *Good Vibrations*, Piatkus Books 1992.

Suzie Hayman, *Hysterectomy*, Sheldon Press 1991.

Suzie Hayman, *Well Woman Handbook*, Penguin Books 1989.

Julia R. Heiman and Joseph LoPiccolo, *Becoming Orgasmic*, Piatkus Books 1988.

Sheila Kitzinger, *Woman's Experience of Sex*, Penguin Books 1983.

Dr Christine E. Sandford, *Enjoy Sex in the Middle Years*, Macdonald Optima 1990.

Yosh Taguchi, *Private Parts*, Macdonald Optima 1988.

Dr Warwick Williams, *It's Up to You*, Thorsons 1989.

Index